AF737013

Perinatal Mental Health and the Military Family

This multi-disciplinary resource provides an overview of perinatal mental and physical health issues within the military population. Perinatal mental health has far-reaching implications for military readiness. The text provides insights into the effects of military culture on identification, evaluation, and treatment of perinatal mood and anxiety disorders and is an invaluable resource for military and civilian primary and behavioral health providers.

Melinda A. Thiam, MD, is a staff psychiatrist in the military where she works as a clinic chief in behavioral health.

Perinatal Mental Health and the Military Family

Identifying and Treating Mood and Anxiety Disorders

Edited by Melinda A. Thiam, MD

Routledge
Taylor & Francis Group
NEW YORK AND LONDON

First published 2017
by Routledge
605 Third Avenue, New York, NY 10017

and by Routledge
2 Park Square, Milton Park, Abingdon, Oxon, OX14 4RN

Routledge is an imprint of the Taylor & Francis Group, an informa business

© 2017 Taylor & Francis

The right of Melinda A. Thiam to be identified as the author of the editorial material, and of the contributors for their individual chapters, has been asserted in accordance with sections 77 and 78 of the Copyright, Designs and Patents Act 1988.

All rights reserved. No part of this book may be reprinted or reproduced or utilised in any form or by any electronic, mechanical, or other means, now known or hereafter invented, including photocopying and recording, or in any information storage or retrieval system, without permission in writing from the publishers.

Trademark notice: Product or corporate names may be trademarks or registered trademarks, and are used only for identification and explanation without intent to infringe.

Library of Congress Cataloging in Publication Data
Names: Thiam, Melinda A., editor.
Title: Perinatal mental health and the military family : identifying and treating mood and anxiety disorders / edited by Melinda A. Thiam.
Description: New York, NY : Routledge, 2016. Includes bibliographical references and index.
Identifiers: LCCN 2016022946 | ISBN 9781138924772 (hbk : alk. paper) | ISBN 9781138924789 (pbk : alk. paper) | ISBN 9781315674858 (ebk)
Subjects: | MESH: Depression, Postpartum—psychology | Depression, Postpartum—therapy | Military Family—psychology | Mothers—psychology | Perinatal Care | Military Psychiatry
Classification: LCC RG852 NLM WQ 500 DDC 618.7/6—dc23
LC record available at https://lccn.loc.gov/2016022946

ISBN: 978-1-138-92477-2 (hbk)
ISBN: 978-1-138-92478-9 (pbk)
ISBN: 978-1-315-67485-8 (ebk)

I am a military service member (or employee of the U.S. Government). This work was prepared as part of my official duties. Title 17, USC, §105 Provides that 'Copyright protection under this title is not available for Any work of the U.S. Government.' Title 17, USC, §101 defines a U.S. Government work as a work prepared by a military service member or Employee of the U.S. Government as part of that person's official duties.

Typeset in Bembo
by Apex CoVantage, LLC

Disclosure

The opinions expressed in this book are those of the authors alone and not necessarily the opinions of the United States Government, United States Army, Department of Defense, United States Navy or Defense Health Agency.

Note: The authors have worked to ensure that all information in this book is accurate at the time of publication and consistent with general psychiatric and medical standards and that information concerning drug dosages, schedules, and routes of administration is accurate at the time of publication and consistent with standards set by the U.S. Food and Drug Administration and the general medical community. As medical research and practice continue to advance, however, therapeutic standards may change. Moreover, specific situations may require a specific therapeutic response not included in this book. For these reasons and because human and mechanical errors sometimes occur, we recommend that readers follow the advice of physicians directly involved in their care or the care of a member of their family.

Contents

Figures

Tables

Foreword

The current world political and economic conditions are evidence that we are living in dangerous times that require increased use of military forces to preserve freedom. Increased demand on military forces will lead to continued stress and demand on troops as they serve in this country, abroad in other countries, and abroad in the deployed environment. In addition to recognizing the tremendous sacrifice of our service members, we must also realize that, along with men and women in uniform, there are countless family members supporting them. The strength of our troops is dependent on the families that support them. Military families are made up of young men and women from a myriad of different backgrounds. Military service members and their families have to cope with stressors of military lifestyle, and there are increasing amounts of behavioral health disorders in service members and their families. Mental health challenges in service members and their spouses have negative effects on the military child, from infancy through adolescence.

In the same fashion, perinatal mood and anxiety disorders have a ripple effect across families and the mental health of parents during pregnancy and early childhood years can have lasting influence on infant/child development. Because military families fall into the age demographic of first-time parenthood, it is critical to examine the effect of perinatal mental health in military families. Both perinatal mental illnesses in the general population and mental health in military families can have consequences if left unrecognized.

There is relatively little literature and research dedicated to discussing perinatal mental health and the military family. This book initially started with a military psychiatry resident trying to improve access to care and provide treatment to a unique subset of the military family that was under-recognized in the literature. As this project progressed, different research from various specialties started to allow for networking between many clinicians who are contributing authors to this text. From this collaboration came a concerted effort by military and civilian providers both inside and outside of the military health system coming together to advocate for the military family. As most authors contributing to this process work for the Department of Defense, there was no compensation, meaning authors volunteered time, knowledge and clinical/academic expertise to produce this manuscript. Providers from the obstetrical field, pediatrics, primary care and behavioral health have all graciously collaborated to produce a multi-disciplinary book that is targeted toward primary care and specialty behavioral health providers to use as a resource for understanding perinatal mood and anxiety disorders, especially within the military population.

As you read this guide, it is broken down to a stepwise fashion. First, we give a review of perinatal mental health, followed by an introduction to the military family and discussion of mental health challenges innate to the military family. Then, we combine these two areas to address perinatal mental health in the military, discussing how military culture and military family dynamics affect the identification, evaluation and treatment of perinatal mood and anxiety disorders. While there has been national effort to move towards collaborative care, perinatal mental health remains under–recognized in both the military and civilian sectors. It is our goal that one day there will be a perinatal mental health network wherein both military health care as well as civilian network providers can come together to provide collaborate health care for service members and their families. It is an honor to dedicate this manuscript to two of the fields near and dear to my heart: the military family and perinatal mental health.

Melinda A. Thiam, MD

Contributors

Melinda A. Thiam, MD, MAJ, USA MC, is a board-certified staff psychiatrist in the military, where she works as a clinic chief in behavioral health, serving active duty military service members and their families at Ft. Jackson, SC. Dr. Thiam enlisted in the MN Army National Guard as an Army medic when she was 17 years old, then transitioned from National Guard to Army ROTC and completed her undergraduate degree with a BS in Biology at Pacific Lutheran University, Tacoma, Washington. She received her medical degree from the Uniform Services University (USUHS) medical school. She completed an internship in pediatrics and then served for a short period as a General Medical Officer at Ft. Lewis, Washington, before switching to psychiatry. During her psychiatry residency, Dr. Thiam designed, led and implemented a mother–infant dyadic therapy group that she co-facilitated for the last 2 years of her residency. Dr. Thiam presented two separate abstracts on perinatal mental health as well as sat on the panel on perinatal mental health and the military family at the American Psychiatric Association annual meeting in 2014. Her research interests include women's mental health, integrated care, complementary/alternative treatment modalities and special topics in military psychiatry.

Rachel M. Bjerstedt, MBA, this book's copyeditor and graphic designer, obtained her MBA from the University of Phoenix. She has been working as a freelance graphic designer, copywriter, and digital marketing consultant for the last 10 years.

Nicole Champagne, LCSW, works at the Naval Medical Center San Diego, NMCSD, in the OB/GYN Department. She received her BS in psychology from Virginia Commonwealth University and MSW from Smith College School for Social Work. Nicole is the co-developer and facilitator of the Perinatal Support Group at NMCSD. In addition, Nicole teaches a Mind-Body-Medicine class to Mothers-to-Be, who are interested in increasing resiliency to stress. Her early experience was working in adoptions for 10 years at a county agency. She is the mother of one son and loves finding ways to benefit her clients that are outside the norm.

Ashley Clark, MD, is a board-certified psychiatrist at the Naval Medical Center San Diego (NMCSD), serving active duty service members, dependents and retirees. Dr. Clark received her BA in human biology from Stanford University and then went on to achieve her medical degree from the University of Vermont, College of Medicine. She completed her internship and residency at Harbor-UCLA Medical Center. During her final year of residency, she served as chief resident and also completed an outpatient program devoted to assessing and treating women with psychiatric conditions associated with hormonal challenges and reproductive life events at the Women's Life Center at the David Geffen School of Medicine at UCLA. Since completing her residency training in psychiatry, Dr. Clark has been a staff psychiatrist at both NMCSD and the San Diego County Psychiatric Hospital. She also serves as the Assistant Program Director for the NMCSD Psychiatry Residency Program. Dr. Clark has also been on the board of the nonprofit organization, Postpartum Health Alliance, for the past five years. She recently attained a second board certification in addiction medicine and continues to enjoy treating patients with a variety of psychiatric conditions.

Amy De Nardo-Kaczmarek, MA, NCC/CCMHC, LPC, served four years as an enlisted soldier in the United States Army from 1999 to 2003 as a mental health specialist and medic. She earned an associate's degree in social sciences with an emphasis in psychology from Brookdale College in 2005. Within less than a year, she earned her bachelor's degree in psychology from Thomas Edison State College in 2006. In 2008, she graduated with a master's degree in professional counseling from South University and was top of her class. In 2011, she passed the National Counseling Exam and became a Licensed Professional Counselor Intern for 2 years, until she was fully licensed as a Professional Counselor in 2013. She took the National Clinical Mental Health Counseling Exam in 2015 and passed. She is a National Certified Counselor and is certified in Scream Free Parenting and Marriage Counseling. In addition to her military service and educational accomplishments, she has worked at a state psychiatric hospital with chronic and acute patients for three years and has worked for the military as a civilian for over four years. She has been married to a military soldier for over 15 years and has two special needs children.

Michael M. Dickman, DO, MAJ, USA MC, is a board-certified family medicine physician and chief of the Soldier Centered Medical Homes at Schofield Barracks, Hawaii, where he works serving active duty military service members. Dr. Dickman received his BA in biology from LaSalle University and went on to graduate medical school from the University of New England College of Osteopathic Medicine in Maine and entered service with the U.S. Army through the Armed Forces Health Professions Scholarship Program. He completed his residency in family medicine at Dewitt Army Community Hospital in Fort Belvoir, Virginia, and has since served military service members and their families on three continents.

Lisa M. Edwards, PhD, is an associate professor in the department of Counselor Education and Counseling Psychology at Marquette University. Dr. Edwards is the Director of Counselor Education and teaches courses in multicultural counseling, group counseling, assessment, and supervision. She directs the Culture and Well-Being Research Lab and is a licensed psychologist in the state of Wisconsin. Dr. Edwards's research focuses on strengths and positive functioning among ethnic minority youth and adults. Specifically, she investigates how cultural variables such as familism, religiosity and ethnic identity influence well-being among Latino/as and multiracial populations. She also studies perinatal mental health and currently works with pregnant and postpartum Latina mothers in Milwaukee. Dr. Edwards is co-author of *Preventing Adolescent Depression and Suicide among Latinas* (2013, Springer Briefs in Psychology) and co-editor of *Perspectives on the Intersection of Multiculturalism and Positive Psychology* (2014, Springer Science+Media).

Kelly O. Elmore, MD, CDR USN, MC, is a native of Chicago, Illinois, who graduated Summa Cum Laude with a bachelor of science degree from Xavier University of Louisiana. Upon completing her medical degree from the University of Chicago, Pritzker School of Medicine, she entered the naval service in 1998 through the Armed Forces Health Professions Scholarship Program. She completed her obstetrics and gynecology internship and residency at the Naval Medical Center San Diego. Between these training programs, she completed a tour as a General Medical Officer at Naval Hospital Roosevelt Roads in Puerto Rico.

While in residency, CDR Elmore presented original research on Group Beta Streptococcus antibiotic resistance at the Armed Forces District annual meeting in Germany. As staff at Naval Hospital Camp Pendleton (NHCP), she co-authored research on the prevalence of peripartum depression, which was presented at the 2011 Academic Research Competition and published in the October 2012 *Journal of Military Medicine.* During her tenure at NHCP, CDR Elmore was the Interim and Assistant Department Head of Obstetrics and Gynecology, the Chair of the NHCP Perinatal Advisory Board, Medical Liaison for Labor and Delivery, as well as the lead women's health consultant for the Johns Hopkins University Applied Sciences Lab OBGYN Process Improvement Project.

Eric M. Flake, MD, LtCol, USAF MC, is the program director of the Department of Defense Developmental Behavioral Pediatrics Fellowship at Joint Base Lewis McChord, Tacoma, Washington. He attended the military medical school (USUHS), graduating in 2001. Dr. Flake is board certified both in pediatrics and developmental and behavioral pediatrics. Dr. Flake has both spoken and published various articles regarding the psychosocial effects of deployment on children. He is an assistant professor at the Uniform Services University and clinical professor at the University of Washington. He is the past-president of the of the Uniformed Services Chapter East for the American Academy of Pediatrics (AAP) and is a member of the science advisory board for the Military Child Education Coalition.

Sharon Gerdes, BSN, CFS, is an author, motivational speaker, and Certified Food Scientist. She is the Health and Wellness editor for *Dairy Foods* magazine. She is the author of over 70 nonfiction articles and a contributing author to four nonfiction books on food, nutrition, childcare and health topics. She speaks internationally on nutrition topics with a focus on the role of protein in muscle synthesis and weight management. She has served as a Senior Account Manager for the U.S. Dairy Export Council, working with major multi-national corporations to design and launch protein-enhanced foods for sports nutrition and weight management. A postpartum psychosis survivor, she volunteers as PR/Marketing Chair and Vice-President of Postpartum Support International (PSI), a nonprofit organization that serves women in 50 states and over 40 countries. She currently hosts a *Food and Mood* blog and is a guest blogger for PSI. She has a BS in Foods and Nutrition from Kansas State University. An avid hiker, she lives in Colorado with her husband of 40 years, a retired Air Force and commercial pilot.

Kellie Haworth, MD, MAJ, USAR, MC, is a board-certified pediatrician and board eligible pediatric hematologist/oncologist currently focusing on research of pediatric malignancy immunologic profiling related to oncolytic virotherapy at Nationwide Children's Hospital in Columbus, Ohio. She is an American Academy of Pediatrics (AAP) fellow and member of their Uniformed Services section and serves as Chair Coordinator for Military Families for Postpartum Support International. Dr. Haworth received her bachelor's degree from Indiana Wesleyan University and medical degree from the Chicago Medical School as a United States Army Health Professions Scholar. She completed pediatric residency training at East Carolina University Brody School of Medicine, then served four years active duty, including interim roles as Chief of Pediatrics and Officer in Charge, at Ireland Army Community Hospital, Fort Knox, Kentucky. Doctor Haworth was honored as the AAP's Uniformed Services Chapter East 2009 "Outstanding Young Pediatrician," and received the Commander's Coin of Excellence for "Exceptionally High Quality of Care" at Fort Knox. She earned first place in the AAP's 2010 Leo J. Geppert Research competition for her research, "Incidence and Severity of Postpartum Depression Among Military Beneficiaries."

She presented "Diapers and Delirium: A Pediatrician's Perspective on Postpartum Depression" at East Carolina University's 2011 Tingelstad conference and offered "Dog Tags and Depression: Addressing the Needs of Military Families" at Postpartum Support International's 2011 meeting. She delivered "Dog Tags, Diapers, and Despair: Addressing Peripartum Needs of Military Families" for the 12th Veteran's Integrated Service Network's Women's Mental Health Mini-Residency in 2014.

David S. Hodson, EdD, APRN, PMHCNS-BC, was born and raised in London, Ontario, earned his baccalaureate degree in nursing from Texas Christian University and his master's degree from Texas Women's University and subsequently earned his doctorate in educational leadership from University of Sarasota. He served as the assistant dean in the School of Nursing at the University of South Carolina. He has worked in nursing and behavioral health care since 1976 and published his master's thesis and doctoral dissertation on nurses' knowledge and attitudes toward electrical convulsive therapy (ECT). He has served as president of the *Alpha Xi* chapter of *Sigma Theta Tau*, in addition to serving as president of the Psychiatric Chapter of the South Carolina Nurses Association. He has facilitated numerous lectures and psychiatric content material for the state of South Carolina, nationally and internationally. He currently serves in the United States Army and as a member of the Department of Defense to preserve the fighting strength of the military and the health of their family.

Valerie Jobrack, MA, LMFT, is a military spouse and Licensed Marriage and Family Therapist. She graduated from John F. Kennedy University with a MA in counseling psychology with a specialization in marriage and family therapy in 2009. She is a 2005 graduate of California State University, Chico, where she earned a bachelor's degree in psychology. As a clinician, Valerie has worked with a variety of clientele, including couples, children and adolescents, and individuals. She is particularly interested in postpartum mood and anxiety disorders and has been the Postpartum Support International Volunteer Coordinator for the United States Air Force branch since 2011.

Daniel J. Lee, MD, MAJ, USA MC, completed his bachelor's degree at DeSales University with foci in biology, psychology and neuroscience. He was commissioned in the US Army and completed his doctorate of medicine at the Uniformed Services University of the Health Sciences. Following medical school, Dr. Lee completed his residency in psychiatry at Walter Reed National Military Medical Center. Following residency, he was assigned to Bayne-Jones Army Community Hospital at Fort Polk, LA. During this assignment, Dr. Lee served in the roles of staff psychiatrist, behavioral health consultant for primary care, chief of the traumatic brain injury, child and family behavioral health service, non-brigade combat team embedded behavioral health, and multi-disciplinary clinics, and served on several committees dealing with management of polypharmacy, controlled substances, and psychoactive substances. He currently works on VA/DoD behavioral health policy and research at the Office of Evidence-Based Medicine at Fort Sam Houston, TX. His research interests/areas of expertise include military medicine, military psychiatry, screening and treatment for posttraumatic stress disorder, treatment refractory mood disorders and treatment refractive posttraumatic stress disorder psychoactive substances, drug–drug interactions, athletic supplements, weight loss supplements, energy supplements, bias assessment, meta-analysis, and research design.

Carla W. Schnitzlein, MD, MAJ USA MC, is a native of Massachusetts who completed undergraduate and medical school in Florida, then graduating from Lake Erie College of Osteopathic Medicine with honors in 2010. She completed her residency at Walter Reed National Military Medical Center in 2014 and is currently a board-certified psychiatrist for the United States Military. Her areas of interest in regards to research are pharmacology and gender studies.

Daniel B. Singley, PhD, is a San Diego-based board-certified psychologist and Director of the Center for Men's Excellence. His research and practice focus on men's mental health with a particular emphasis on reproductive psychology and the transition to fatherhood. He conducts trainings and presentations around the country to assist individuals and organizations to enhance their level of father inclusiveness and founded the grant-funded Basic Training for New Dads, Inc., nonprofit in order to give new fathers the tools they need to be highly engaged with their infants, as well as their partners. He is past-president of the APA's Section on Positive Psychology and currently serves on the Boards of the APA's Division on the Psychological Study of Men and Masculinity as well as Postpartum Support International.

Sondra S. Thompson, MSN, APRN, PMHCNS-BC, is an advanced practice registered nurse who has worked in the military psychiatric setting for more than 25 years. She retired from the United States Army Nurse Corps after a total of 25 years consisting of both enlisted and officer service. She completed her undergraduate degree in nursing at the University of North Carolina, Greensboro, and her master's degree in nursing at the University of Colorado Health Sciences Center. She has presented on topics of stress effects and management and provider self-care. She is particularly interested in "care of the caregivers" to assist health care providers in dealing with the demands of giving so much in providing treatment. As a veteran of Operation Iraqi Freedom herself, she finds that her greatest passion and honor is that of providing care for the military and their families throughout the demands of military service. She is currently enjoying life after active duty, sailing as often as possible and continues to work with the military at Fort Jackson, South Carolina in the Department of Behavioral Health at Moncrief Army Community Hospital.

Karen L. Weis, PhD, RNC, FAAN, is Professor and Endowed Chair of Nursing at the University of the Incarnate Word. She accepted this appointment after retiring from the United States Air Force after 28 years on active duty. During this time, she served as dean of the Medical Education and Training Campus, where over 6,500 students a day from the Army, Navy and Air Force are educated and trained in over 47 enlisted medical career fields. Before this assignment, she was the dean of the United States Air Force School of Aerospace Medicine, where she was responsible for the education and training of both enlisted and officers in public health, bioenvironmental, aerospace physiology, and flight medicine. Dr. Weis holds a master's degree in high-risk obstetrical nursing and her doctoral emphasis and continued research are in the areas of maternal identity formation and adaptation to pregnancy. She has been the primary investigator for over $1.5 million in funded research and has published primarily in the field of prenatal maternal psychosocial health. She co-authored the third edition of the *Psychosocial Adaptation to Pregnancy: Seven Dimensions of Maternal Role Development.*

Part I

Introduction to Perinatal Mental Health

Chapter 1

The Psychological Aspects of Motherhood

Melinda A. Thiam, Kelly O. Elmore, and Karen L. Weis

In the course of becoming a mother, a woman psychologically transitions into a mindset of a mother as she adapts from a known, current reality to an unknown, new reality (Stern & Bruschweiler-Stern, 1998). This transition to motherhood requires a mother to restructure her goals, behaviors and responsibilities to develop a new sense of self, which is termed the "motherhood identity" (Mercer, 2004).

The motherhood identity orginates in early childhood when girls first act out societal gender roles while playing (Stern & Bruschweiler-Stern, 1998). At this age, girls are still in early stages of developing their sense of self as male or female, and they perceive/label certain activities and forms of play as belonging to a particular gender (Stern & Bruschweiler-Stern, 1998). For example, girls may participate in "feminine" forms of pretend play such as "house" or dress up or playing with dolls. In contrast, boys engage in "masculine" activities that are usually physical in nature. From these forms of play, children will eventually incorporate cultural and societal influences into their gender identity that will affect how they perceive social and interpersonal roles.

Motivations and Beliefs About Motherhood

Overview

In many cultures around the world, from first-world countries to third-world countries, motherhood is a socially prescribed role. Many of these countries see motherhood and the experience of motherhood vital to being seen as a "wholly functioning woman" (Boucai & Karniol, 2008). Even during childhood, various cultures across the world directly or indirectly imply that becoming a wife and mother defines the female role and is essential to female identity (Boucai & Karniol, 2008). Due to this social expectation of motherhood, it is genuinely not socially acceptable for women to express a lack of a desire for a child (Boucai & Karniol, 2008). As a result, women who remain childless, regardless of reason, may experience internal and external stigma.

Traditionally, motherhood was seen as a woman's full-time job and primary responsibility; mothers were not supposed to engage in work outside of the home (Boucai & Karniol, 2008). In this modern area, the expansion of gender equality enables women to participate in a wide array of careers and pursue numerous employment opportunities as they are now culturally "liberated" and able to play social roles other than "just" motherhood. Some women elect to focus primarily on careers, some women choose to work in the home full time, while other women will simultaneously pursue both roles as working mothers. Many women embrace this opportunity to pursue both a career and experience motherhood. Working mothers are valued members in the workplace and frequently can pursue motherhood and career advancement. On the other hand, women who pursue work and motherhood still experience the internal societal "expectation of motherhood." Women who pursue career option may still subconsciously struggle with this expectation of motherhood, which can lead to a role conflict resulting in women feeling that they must make a choice, between work or motherhood.

Interpersonal role conflict in addressing the beliefs about work and motherhood became a hot topic in the media in 2002, when Oprah Winfrey hosted an episode titled "Motherhood Wars" (Johnston & Swanson, 2004). In this nationally televised episode, two psychologists argued on opposing sides about the ability of mothers to fulfill dual roles of being both a mother and a member of the workforce (Johnston & Swanson, 2004). The "Motherhood Wars" episode became a media sensation and brought public awareness to society's conflicting beliefs about mothers' decision to stay home versus return to work (Johnston & Swanson, 2004). Dr. Laura Schlessinger argued for the traditional motherhood role inside the home and emphatically stated that women who work should not be parents, because, by pursuing a career, a woman neglects her mothering duties. On the opposing side, Dr. Peters argued for mothers working outside the home and stated that women who do so are better, more well-adjusted mothers (Johnston & Swanson, 2004). Although these providers represent polarized views on what it means to be a "good mother," it was discovered that women usually approved of other individuals who made the same work/motherhood choice they did. Socially, women may feel that other women who made a different choice are "not good mothers"(Johnston & Swanson, 2004). This research found that regardless of their choice, many women still felt unsupported by the culture (Johnston & Swanson, 2004), and gender-role stereotypes remain pervasive. No matter what type of role a woman pursues, she may find herself at odds with culture (Miner, Pesonen, Smittick, Clark, & Seigel, 2014). Women who remain childless may be perceived as selfish, competitive and pursuing male gender roles (Miner et al., 2014). Working mothers are accused of depriving their children of a mom and being incapable of balancing professional goals and expectations (Miner et al., 2014). In contrast, mothers who stay at home may be seen as individuals who gave up their careers and identities in the workforce to become "just a mother" who obtained domestic success but are incapable of achieving success outside the home (Johnston & Swanson, 2004).

To Work or to Stay Home, That Is the Question

The number of mothers engaging in the workforce has nearly doubled from 47% in 1975 to 71% in 2008 (Miner et al., 2014). Despite more equal opportunity employment, employed mothers face a myriad of obstacles, most often secondary to stereotyping and discrimination regarding gender in the workplace (Miner et al., 2014). Employed mothers were found to have lower wages, lower likelihood of being hired, lower likelihood of being promoted, and were often perceived as having less competence and dedication compared to their male peers (Miner et al., 2014). Despite these challenges, many mothers still choose to work outside the home and are satisfied with their decision (Miner et al., 2014). Ultimately, the decision to return to work after delivery is an individual decision that a woman makes depending on her financial situation, personal desires, cultural expectations and beliefs regarding parenting.

Transition to Motherhood

Although the initial process of the motherhood identity begins in childhood, the process of "becoming a mother" begins at conception and continues after her child is born (Stern & Bruschweiler-Stern, 1998). The motherhood identity that began in childhood will remain dormant until awakened once a woman discovers that she is pregnant (Stern & Bruschweiler-Stern, 1998). The process of becoming a mother has been described in four stages: acceptance of pregnancy and commitment to the maternal role; "meeting" the baby and starting to physically/emotional engage in active tasks of motherhood; adjusting to social roles; and the establishment of her maternal identity (Mercer, 2004). Maternal identity formation requires a woman to relinquish former physical, mental and social self and adapt to pregnancy and postpartum changes in physical, mental and social aspects (Weis, 2006). We will describe these aspects of the transition to motherhood using a biopsychosocial model, beginning with physiological and concluding with cultural/religious issues.

Biological and Physical Changes in Becoming a Mother

Pregnancy is an inherently disruptive physiological process due to the significant physical, hormonal, neurochemical and neurobiological shifts that occur within the body of a pregnant woman (Slade, Cohen, Sadler, & Miller, 2009). A woman has to adapt to physical changes of varying degrees throughout her pregnancy and then return to baseline after birth in the postpartum period.

Pregnancy requires a woman to maintain health for the sake of herself and her developing fetus. During pregnancy, women become cognizant of health behaviors and may engage in behavioral changes such as quitting smoking, abstaining from alcohol or being more mindful of actions/situations harmful to health.

From Conception to the First Trimester

Pregnancy ultimately begins at conception; from the moment of conception, a cascade of physical, biological and neural changes can be detected within days of fertilization of the ovum followed by beginning stages of an embryo (Slade et al., 2009). The greatest amount of development occurs within the first 12 weeks of pregnancy, also known as the first trimester. (Slade et al., 2009). During the first trimester, the developing fetus is most vulnerable to toxic influences (Slade et al., 2009). The first trimester is critical for the development of organs and nervous system, yet, many women remain unaware of their pregnancy until halfway through this trimester. During these early stages of pregnancy, an expectant mother undergoes a myriad of physical changes. There are multiple hormonal, cardiovascular, neuroendocrine, respiratory, musculoskeletal, hair/skin and nail changes during pregnancy (Foley, 2014). Typical symptoms of early pregnancy include amenorrhea, nausea (with/without vomiting), breast enlargement and tenderness, increased frequency of urination and fatigue (Bastian & Brown, 2014).

Second and Third Trimester

The second trimester is a time of significant fetal growth, a time when a woman typically feels her baby move for first time and when she begins to "feel" pregnant (Slade et al, 2009). The second trimester is also when a woman usually discovers the gender of her child. Along with progression in fetal development, a pregnant mother also experiences musculoskeletal changes, weight gain, water retention and hormone changes that occur to accommodate for the growing fetus (Bastian & Brown, 2014).

In the third trimester, the baby is almost fully developed, and mothers gain the greatest amount of weight during this time (Slade et al., 2009). Women begin to prepare for birth and often describe being incredibly fatigued. The third trimester is also the time when woman's body prepares for physical challenges of labor. She may struggle with sleep, and the size of the fetus can make moving around and participating in daily activities more difficult.

Birth and Postpartum Recovery

After birth, a woman's body undergoes significant physiological shifts so it can return to its baseline state. Soon after delivery, there is a rapid change in hormones, leading to a sudden drop in estrogen and progesterone. These abrupt hormone changes have been theorized to predispose to development of postpartum depression or anxiety. In addition to the internal physiological changes that affect recovery from pregnancy, there are also external biological factors such as nutritionally balanced diet, adequate sleep and environmental stressors.

Psychological Changes

Psychoanalyst Dr. Daniel Stern describes the psychological transition to motherhood as a psychological process that parallels the physical changes that occur in pregnancy (Stern & Bruschweiler-Stern, 1998). The psychological process of becoming a mother requires a woman to transition from a known reality and interpersonal social role to the unknown new role. This developmental transition requires a mother to restructure her goals, behaviors and responsibilities so she can transition to development of her new sense of self (Mercer, 2004).

Acceptance of Pregnancy

During the first trimester of gestation, an expectant mother must come to accept the idea of being pregnant (Weis, 2006). Acceptance of pregnancy is a crucial component of a woman's adaptation to pregnancy and beginning of maternal identity formation (Weis, Lederman, Lilly, & Schaffer, 2008). During the first trimester, women may experience some internal ambivalence as they balance the idea of a child with the subjective experience of becoming a mother (Weis et al., 2008). By the time women reach the second trimester, women have usually accepted the pregnancy and have committed to the maternal role (Weis, 2006).

Women with challenging social circumstances, such as being a single parent, or being separated from their from family or primary support network, may struggle to accept their pregnancy. Women who refuse to accept their pregnancies may resent being pregnant and remain detached from all aspects of pregnancy (Stern & Bruschweiler-Stern, 1998). Fortunately, the 9-month duration of pregnancy allows most mothers time to resolve internal dissonance related to undesired pregnancy, and the majority of women will eventually be able to accept their role as a mother (Lederman & Weis, 2009).

Expectations

Expectations of pregnancy and hope of motherhood can affect a woman's ability to adapt to psychological transition to motherhood. In pregnancy, women often have expectations of what pregnancy will be like (Weis et al., 2008). Women who experience undesired/unexpected physical changes may become internally distressed, as this experience goes against their expectation; on the other hand, women who expect to feel miserable, but do not experience such, may also feel distressed (Weis et al., 2008).

Expectations of what it is like to be a mother often begin in childhood and become more active during pregnancy (Stern & Bruschweiler-Stern, 1998). Many women have inaccurate or unrealistic expectations of motherhood that are based on experiences of their friends or their mothers (Ambrosini & Stanghellini, 2012; Weaver & Ussher, 1997). Women may base their views about motherhood on traditional images of attractive/perfectly dressed and made-up mothers with happy, smiling families (Weaver & Ussher, 1997). After birth, many first-time mothers discover motherhood is very different from their imagined perspective on motherhood. (Barnes & Balber, 2007; Weaver & Ussher, 1997). When mothers do not meet their lofty expectation of motherhood, they experience what has been described as the "myth of motherhood" (Weaver & Ussher, 1997). Women who feel let down by unmet expectations may subsequently feel distraught with motherhood as they face the new role and job description, not feeling competent or confident in their ability to parent (Barnes & Balber, 2007).

Personality, Cognitive Flexibility, and Confidence

A woman's personality and cognitive flexibility can influence how she experiences motherhood. Mothers who have rigid thinking processes struggle with aspects of motherhood when they do not feel that they are in control of the process. Women who feel they are not in control of their pregnancy, labor or delivery process are at increased risk of distress and may experience difficulty transitioning to motherhood (Buultjens & Liamputtong, 2007). For instance, once a mother brings her child home, she enters into a realm where she may not feel confident or competent, especially if other individuals challenge her parenting skills or give unsolicited/unwanted advice (Stern & Bruschweiler-Stern, 1998).

Transition in Dyadic Interpersonal Relationships

A "dyadic" relationship describes a one-on-one relationship between two people (Shea, 1998). The two most significant dyadic relationships in the transition to motherhood are the mother–infant dyad and the marital dyad (or relationship with significant other).

The Mother–Infant Dyad

The mother–infant dyad is one of the primary relationships that forms the foundation of the mother–baby bond and will subsequently influence the trajectory of her infant's attachment. The mother–infant relationship begins prenatally and will influence her ability to bond with her infant after birth. During pregnancy, a mother begins to fanaticize or wonder about her baby's personality (Slade et al., 2009). In the process of this wondering about her baby, a woman may unconsciously project her ambitions and subconscious wishes unto her unborn child (Stern & Bruschweiler-Stern, 1998). The development of the mother–infant bond will be further explored in Chapter 3 on infant mental health.

The Marital Dyad: Adjusting Marital Roles

Pregnancy is also a time of changing roles in relationships and will require changes in the marital relationship as both expectant parents prepare for parenthood (Lederman & Weis, 2009). Preparation for parenthood begins in pregnancy. Both future parents will need to examine their unresolved conflicts from childhood, as well as recognize how their individual childhood experiences may influence how they view their parenting role. It is crucial for an expectant couple to recognize that becoming parents will change the dynamics of their marriage: conflicts frequently occur when parents do not plan for or acknowledge that there will be significant changes in their relationship (Barnes & Balber, 2007).

Future parents should discuss the significance of various family transitions, as well as beliefs about the traditional roles in parenting. The two most common parental role perspectives are the *traditional* and *egalitarian* perspectives on individual parental roles. In the traditional role, the mother will usually take responsibility for baby, and the father will see his role relegated to providing support. Husbands' worries may turn outward, while wives' fears and concerns turn inward. For example, mothers may feel pressure to protect their baby's safety and be primarily responsible for their baby's well-being, growth and development. In contrast, a father may feel the need to keep the family safe and financially secure, and thus may experience a mix of confusion, jealousy, wonder and inadequacy as he observes the bond between his wife and child (Barnes & Balber, 2007). The egalitarian perspective often leads to similar roles but recognizes that both parents need to contribute equally to parenting, and the parent–infant bonding is not limited to the mother. Although many societies may outwardly express support of egalitarian perspective, many individuals may consciously or unconsciously internalize traditional gender roles and expectations.

Revisiting Family of Origin: Psychodynamic Aspects of Being Parented

Family of origin has a significant impact on a mother's developmental transition to motherhood. How a woman was raised will influence how she engages in interpersonal relationships and views the world (Stern & Bruschweiler-Stern, 1998). Critical psychological tasks during the transition to motherhood require an expectant mother to revisit or reflect past relationships with her parents. For example, when a woman finds out she will be a mother, she will often consciously or unconsciously recall the relationship she had with her mother—good or bad (Stern & Bruschweiler-Stern, 1998). For instance, a woman may reflect on painful or sad memories about her experience with her mother (Barnes & Balber, 2007). Some women may have unresolved psychological conflict in relationship to their mothers, while others may hope that a bad relationship can be reconciled. Unresolved past trauma from childhood can influence women to reenact such experiences with her infant (Frailberg, Adelson, & Shapiro, 1975; Stern & Bruschweiler-Stern, 1998).

Changes in Group Identity and Interpersonal Roles

Group-interpersonal roles represent how an individual relates to groups of individuals, as opposed to one-on-one (Shea, 1998). The manner in which a mother identifies herself within various social groups will change as she transitions into her motherhood role (Alstveit, Severinsson, & Karlson, 2011). When transitioning to motherhood, women often find themselves seeking the support of other women, especially other mothers, and may feel the urge to swap information and/or observe other mothers in action (Darvill, Skirton, & Farrand, 2010; Stern & Bruschweiler-Stern, 1998). Interactions with other mothers serve as a form of affirmation to help a mother feel confident/competent in her new role. Stern and Bruschweiler conducted a study in Boston wherein they surveyed mothers to determine how much contact these mothers had with people after their baby was born (Stern & Bruschweiler-Stern, 1998). They found that new mothers sought out help from experienced mothers, and in an average day, the new mothers had more than 10 different contacts in the form of visits or telephone calls (Stern & Bruschweiler-Stern, 1998).

Changes in Pre-existing Groups Relationships/Interpersonal Roles

A woman's relationship with her workplace is a "group" relationship (Alstveit et al., 2011). Women who return to work need to learn to adjust to both their role as an employee and their role as a mother (Alstveit et al., 2011; Dagher, Hofferth, & Lee, 2014). New mothers must be able to balance these roles as they learn to manage their workplace workload as well as the best interests of their child (Alstveit et al., 2011). Women learning to find balance in these roles may frequently struggle with feelings of not being a "good enough" mother (Alstveit et al., 2011) and may feel that they are 'failing' at both roles.

Transitions in Societal System

The societal system looks at how economic, political and institutional systems influence an individual (Shea, 1998). Societal influences on the transition to motherhood include logistical and economic considerations. Parenting is expensive, and socio-economic concerns can create a negative connotation on mothering. Mothers struggling to make ends meet and who obtain government assistance through WIC, food stamps or welfare may be viewed as "unfit" mothers due to societal sterotypes and judgment about what may have happened to a women to get into such circumstances, based on what they read in the newspaper or hear in political discussions (Cronin, 2003).

Framework of Meaning

An individual's "framework of meaning" includes an individual's philosophical beliefs, religious beliefs and ethical standards (Shea, 1998). In many cultures, religious/moral beliefs are built off of cultural practices, and there may be particular religious beliefs surrounding motherhood and the postpartum period (Eberhard-Gran, Garthus-Niegel, Garthus-Niegel, & Eskild, 2010).

Different cultures have rites of passage ceremonies to mark transition periods such as pregnancy and childbirth (Eberhard-Gran et al., 2010). Cultures across the world have different customs that occur secondary to viewing the postpartum state as a "rite-of-passage" transition. Many of these customs center around five core concepts: a distinct postpartum period; protective measures and rituals; social seclusion of new mother and mandated rest; assistance from relatives in daily tasks; and social recognition through rituals and gifts to acknowledge the status of the new mother (Eberhard-Gran et al., 2010). Unfortunately, in many countries/religions postpartum rituals are decreasing, and women may now miss the social support, rest and assistance that can facilitate their transition to motherhood. The lack of cultural rituals in the perinatal period can negatively affect a mother's self-esteem, increase stress in marital relationships and increase the likelihood of ambivalence regarding motherhood (Eberhard-Gran et al., 2010).

A woman's religious and philosophical beliefs can also shape how the motherhood role is viewed and how help is sought. Women who have strong religious beliefs benefit from faith-based support. A social support group called Mothers of Preschoolers (MOPS) was created as a faith-based support group for women who wanted to share everyday mothering experiences in a group setting that also included aspects of their faith (Crowley, 2012).

Summary

Pregnant women go through significant biopsychosocial changes in the transition to motherhood. It is important for health care providers treating pregnant and postpartum women to understand how physiological, psychological, interpersonal dyadic and group relationship as well as societal and cultural factors influence the process of becoming a mother. When women struggle with any of these factors when developing their motherhood identity, such struggle can create a context for developing mood or anxiety disorders. In the next chapter, we will discuss what happens when there are disturbances in the physical and psychological transition to motherhood and how these disturbances can lead to mental health disorders.

References

Alstveit, M., Severinsson, E., & Karlson, B. (2011). Readjusting one's life in the tension inherent in work and motherhood. *Journal of Advanced Nursing, 67*(10), 2151–2160.

Ambrosini, A., & Stanghellini, G. (2012). Myths of motherhood: The role of culture in the development of postpartum depression. *Ann Ist Super Sanità, 48*(3), 277–286.

Barnes, D., & Balber, L. (2007). *The Journey to Parenthood: Myths, Realities and What Really Matters.* Oxon, UK: Radcliffe Publishing.

Bastian, L., & Brown, H. (2014). *Clinical Manifestations and Diagnosis of Early Pregnancy.* In: UpToDate, Post TW (Ed), UpToDate, Waltham, MA. (Accessed on June, 2015). Retrieved from www.uptodate.com

Boucai, L., & Karniol, R. (2008). Suppressing and priming the motivation for motherhood. *Sex Roles, 59*, 851–870.

Buultjens, M., & Liamputtong, P. (2007). When giving life starts to take the life out of you: Women's experiences of depression after childbirth. *Midwifery, 23*, 77–91.

Cronin, C. (2003). First-time mothers—identifying their needs, perceptions and experiences. *Journal of Clinical Nursing, 12*, 260–267.

Crowley, J. (2012). Strictly for evangelical parenting support? The case for Mothers of Preschoolers (MOPS). *Review of Religious Research, 54*, 421–444.

Dagher, R., Hofferth, S., & Lee, Y. (2014). Maternal depression, pregnancy intention, and return to paid work after childbirth. *Women's Health Issues, 24*(3), e297–e303.

Darvill, R., Skirton, H., & Farrand, P. (2010). Psychological factors that impact a women's experiences of first-time motherhood: A qualitative study of the transition. *Midwifery, 26*, 357–366.

Eberhard-Gran, M., Garthus-Niegel, S., Garthus-Niegel, K., & Eskild, A. (2010). Postnatal care: A cross-cultural and historical perspective. *Archives of Women's Mental Health, 13*, 459–466.

Foley, M. R. (Producer). (2014). *Maternal Cardiovascular and Hemodynamic Adaptations to Pregnancy.* In: UpToDate, Post TW (Ed), UpToDate, Waltham, MA. (Accessed on June, 2015). Retrieved from http://www.uptodate.com/home/help-manual-citing

Frailberg, S., Adelson, E., & Shapiro, V. (1975). Ghosts in the nursery: A psychoanalytic approach to the problems of impaired infant-mother relationships. *The American Journal of Child Psychiatry, 14*(1–4), 387–421.

Johnston, D., & Swanson, D. (2004). Moms hating moms: The internalization of mother war rhetoric. *Sex Roles, 51*(9–10), 497–509.

Lederman, R., & Weis, K. (2009). *Psychosocial Adaption to Pregnancy: Seven Dimensions of Maternal Role Development.* New York: Springer.

Mercer, R. (2004). Becoming a mother versus maternal role attainment. *Journal of Nursing Scholarship, 36*(3), 719–728.

Miner, K., Pesonen, A., Smittick, A., Clark, E., & Seigel, M. (2014). Does being a mom help or hurt? Workplace incivility as a function of motherhood status. *Journal of Occupational Health Psychology, 19*(1), 60–73.

Shea, S. C. (1998). *Psychiatric Interviewing: The Art of Understanding a Practical Guide for Psychiatrists, Psychologists, Counselors, Social Workers, Nurses, and Other Mental Health Professionals* (2nd ed.). Philadelphia, PA: Saunders.

Slade, A., Cohen, L., Sadler, L., & Miller, M. (2009). The psychology and psychopathology of pregnancy. In C. Zeanah (Ed.), *Handbook of Infant Mental Health* (3rd ed., pp. 22–39). New York: The Guilford Press.

Stern, D., & Bruschweiler-Stern, N. (1998). *The Birth of a Mother: How the Motherhood Experience Changes You Forever.* New York: Basic Books.

Weaver, J., & Ussher, J. (1997). How motherhood changes life—a discourse analytic study with mothers of young children. *Journal of Reproductive & Infant Psychology, 15*(1), 51–68.

Weis, Karen L. (2006). Maternal Identity Formation in a Military Sample: A Longitudal Perspective. Dissertation submitted to University of North Carolina, Chapel Hill.

Weis, Karen L., Lederman, R., Lilly, A., & Schaffer, J. (2008). The relationship of military imposed marital separations on maternal acceptance of pregnancy. *Research in Nursing & Health, 31*, 196–207.

Chapter 2

Overview of Perinatal Mood and Anxiety Disorders

Melinda A. Thiam and Karen L. Weis

Introduction to Perinatal Mood and Anxiety Disorders

Pregnancy was thought to be a time of clinical well-being, however now it has been recognized that depression and other mood disorders can occur in the antepartum period just like they can occur in the postpartum period (Newport, Fernandez, Juric, & Stowe, 2014). Perinatal Mood and Anxiety Disorders (PMADs) are mood and anxiety disorders that occur during pregnancy or up until 1 year postpartum (Indman, Meyer, & Davis, 2013). PMADs have unique characteristics when compared to mood and anxiety disorders that occur during other periods of a woman's life. PMADs have unique physiological and biological basis (O'Hara, Wisner, Asher, & Asher, 2014) and are often accompanied by unique psychological, interpersonal and social changes (see Figure 2.1).

Risk Factors for Perinatal Mood and Anxiety Disorders

Physiological Contributors to Risk

The biological basis of depression has been hypothesized to be secondary to a deficiency in neurotransmitters such as serotonin, dopamine and norepinephrine, as well as the enzyme that breaks down these neurotransmitters (Rechenberg & Humphries, 2013). In additional to neurotransmitter influence, biological underpinnings of perinatal mood and anxiety disorder are affected by dramatic shifts in neuroendocrine hormones such as estrogen and progesterone. These hormones have large increases in levels as the body first adapts to pregnancy followed by sudden drop in hormone levels in postpartum period (Robertson, Celasun, & Stewart, 2003). These hormone levels are closely linked to neurotransmitter levels because estrogen is synergistic with serotonin. Estrogen modulates the serotonin receptor activity and decreased estrogen levels are associated with lower serotonin levels. These hormone fluctuations are thought to destabilize the serotonin system in vulnerable women (O'Hara & McCabe, 2013).

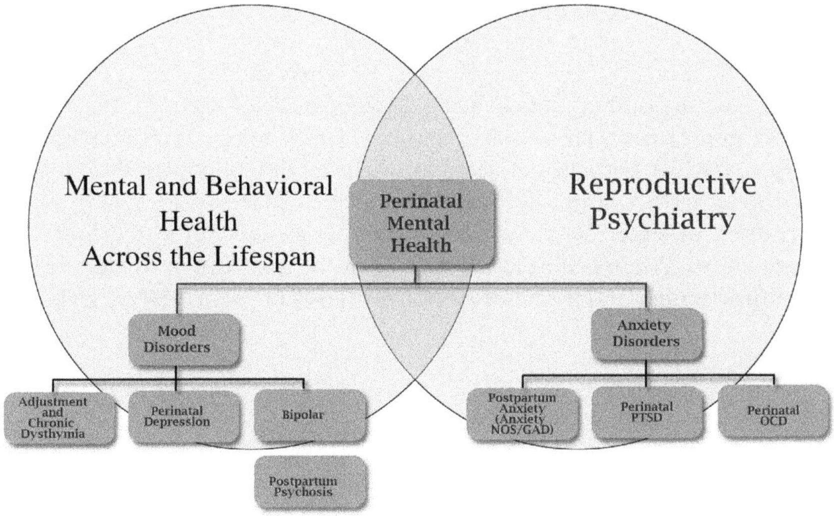

Figure 2.1 Flow Diagram of Perinatal Mood and Anxiety Disorders

Genetic and Past Medical/Psychiatric History

Genetics and family history of mental illness are risk factors for mood and anxiety disorders in the general population as well as perinatal population. Up to 50% of women who experience postpartum depression have a family history of psychiatric illness (Kimmel et al., 2015; National Institute of Health and Care Excellence [NICE], 2014; Williams, 2014). Other medical factors include the history of trauma or loss, unplanned/unwanted pregnancy, birth trauma, difficult/high-risk pregnancy, history of infertility, substance abuse, infertility/history of prior perinatal loss (American Academy of Pediatrics [AAP], 2011).

Sleep Deprivation

Studies have found that insomnia and poor sleep quality/quantity independently increase the risk of depression and anxiety in general populations (Lawson, Murphy, Sloan, Uleryk, & Dalfen, 2015). Likewise, in the perinatal, sleep challenges in pregnant or postpartum women also have negative influence on mood and anxiety. During pregnancy, expectant mothers experience dramatic changes in sleep patterns and women frequently struggle with sleep deprivation due to functional challenges of finding comfortable sleeping position due to changes in body shape. On the other hand, in the postpartum period, sleep deprivation is often secondary to practical tasks of motherhood such as caring for a new infant who usually feeds on demand every 2–4 hours. Postpartum mothers may struggle to sleep when the baby sleeps and feel like they are in constant state of sleep deprivation (Sloan, 2011). Thus, sleep changes in pregnancy are usually secondary to physiological changes during pregnancy, while postpartum sleep disorders are more frequent due to sleep deprivation and nighttime feedings (Verinder & Mazmanian, 2003). Sleep deprivation in either pregnancy or postpartum period can lead to negative consequences. For example, more than 72 hours may lead to impaired cognitive functioning and increases risk of psychosis or mania (Sloan, 2011).

Vitamin D Deficiency

Research has shown a correlation between vitamin D deficiency and an increased risk of depression in individuals in the general population and especially in perinatal population (Polak, Houghton, Reeder, Harper & Conner, 2014; Robinson et al., 2014). Pregnant and postpartum women have an increased likelihood of vitamin D deficiency. Mothers who breastfeed are at increased risk of vitamin D deficiency given increased synthesis of breast milk leads to increased depletion of vitamin D because vitamin D is required in synthesis of breast milk (Polak et al., 2014).

Vitamin D is correlated with mental health secondary to its ability to serve as neurotrophic protective factor (Polak et al., 2014). While vitamin D deficiency is most frequently affected by sun exposure, lower vitamin D levels were still associated with higher depression score even after controlling for confounders such as time spent outdoors (Polak et al., 2014).

Underlying Medical Disorders

Underlying chronic medical illnesses, such as autoimmune diseases, neurological diseases, endocrine diseases and pain disorders, have been correlated with increased rates of depression in the general population. While some women may have pre-existing medical problems when entering pregnancy, the substantial shifts in pregnancy also predispose a woman to developing new disorders or exacerbating current disorders.

Psychological Risk Factors

Psychological risk factors for depression in all periods of life include neuroticism, low self-esteem, rigid cognitive thought processes, guilt/shame, poor coping mechanisms, negative self-image and feelings of helplessness (O'Hara et al., 2014; Robertson et al., 2003; Ward-Zimmerman & Verdetti, 2014). In similar fashion, mothers with depression may feel ashamed and humiliated when they believe they are "failing" at being a mother and come to view themselves as the worst mothers in the world. Such mothers typically assume that others see them in the same way they view themselves (Paris, Bolton, & Weinberg, 2009). Additionally, many women enter pregnancy with false expectations, believing that pregnancy and parenthood will not lead to significant changes. Some of these mothers often take on an extraordinary amount of work and expect to complete all pre-baby tasks and procedures as well as taking care of an infant, keeping the house clean and cooking extravagant meals. A mother's pre-existing perfectionist beliefs may influence her to create unrealistic demands of herself, being overly critical about every mistake she makes, and self-punitive to perceived inadequacies. These beliefs may cause a mother to discount successes and perceive mistakes as devastating (Maia et al., 2012; Robertson et al., 2003).

Body Image/Self-Esteem

Body image and self-esteem can be a particular concern for women with a history of eating disorders or who work in an occupation that values thinness (Downs, DiNallo, & Kirner, 2008). This subject will be discussed in the Appendix.

Dyadic Risk Factors

The particular dyads that become pertinent in perinatal mood and anxiety disorders include the mother–infant dyad (discussed further in the following chapter) and mother–partner dyad. Disruptions in any of these important dyadic relationships may lead to poor bonding, attachment and interactions between mother and infant can lead to distress (Ward-Zimmerman & Verdetti, 2014). Negative changes in marital dyad or relationship with her significant other can lead a woman to feel unsupported during pregnancy and new motherhood (Ward-Zimmerman & Verdetti, 2014).

Group/Societal Risk Factors

Numerous societal factors can predispose a woman to develop perinatal mental illness. One crucial societal factor is the popular media's portrayal of the expected body type, body weight and physical image of pregnant and postpartum women (Gow, Lydecker, Lamanna, & Mazzeo, 2012).

Other social risk factors include poverty/financial hardships, poor/inadequate social support, domestic violence, high levels of childcare stress, teenage motherhood, single motherhood and military service, and maternity and paternity leave policies (AAP, 2011; Ward-Zimmerman & Verdetti, 2014).

The Most Common Perinatal Mood and Anxiety Disorders

Postpartum Blues

Postpartum blues, also known as "baby blues" is the most common type of perinatal distress with some sources citing up to 50% to 80% prevalence in new mothers (Beck, 2006; O'Hara et al., 2014; Williams, 2014). Postpartum blues manifests with a dysphoric mood, anxiety, insomnia, loss of appetite, crying, irritability, fatigue and emotional lability immediately following birth. While many women will recover from this temporary distress, up to 20% of these women will go on to develop postpartum depression (Robertson et al., 2003).

Perinatal Depression

> "I was crying and tired constantly. I had slipped into a sadness that I could not escape. Everything was dark. I felt there was no light at the end of the tunnel. It just seemed to go on and on. I started to feel hopeless as if there was absolutely nothing that could save me from all of this. I became unable to care for my infant daughter and unable to care for myself. I began to think about ways to kill myself. I thought about my children, and what their lives would be like without me. I thought about my husband and figured he'd be better off without me there crying and crazy."
>
> (Submitted to postpartum support international, Military Chapter)

Perinatal depression is a Major Depressive Disorder (MDD) that is temporally associated with depression during pregnancy or the year postpartum (Williams, 2014; Yonkers et al., 2012). Approximately 5%–16% of women will experience depression at some point during their pregnancy, and 4.2%–9.6% will experience depression between birth and 3 months postpartum (Williams, 2014). Antenatal depression occurs in 3%–16% of pregnant women (Gentile, 2011), while postpartum depression occurs in 10%–20% of adult women, and up to 26% of adolescent women (Newport et al., 2014). Perinatal depression is diagnosed clinically, often with support of screening instruments such as Edinburgh Postpartum Depression Scale, EPDS (O'Hara et al., 2014).

A major depressive disorder negatively affects mood, motivation, energy and cognition. Perinatal depression includes the following symptoms: depressed mood or feelings of despair, prominent anxiety, obsessive or compulsive thoughts and irrational fears, feeling out of control of ones thoughts and emotions, feelings of guilt and personal inadequacy, as well as struggling to cope with basic daily tasks (Goodman & Santangelo, 2011; also, see Table 2.1).

Perinatal author and expert Cheryl Beck described perinatal depression as a "thief that steals motherhood" to illustrate how perinatal depression often directly affects a mother's sense of who she is and how she sees herself as a

Table 2.1 How to Distinguish Depression from Normal Mood Swings

Persistent and marked depressed mood
Persistent/marked loss of pleasure (doesn't enjoy interacting with infant)
Feelings of hopelessness
Statements about being a "bad" mother
Feelings of guilt/worthlessness/shame
Withdrawing from friends and family

Source: Adapted from Williams, J. (2014). Best practice guidelines for mental health disorders in the perinatal period. *BC Mental Health.* Retrieved from http://www.perinatalservicesbc.ca/health-professionals/guidelines-standards/maternal 24 January 2016

mother (Beck, 2006). In particular, perinatal depression affects a mother's sense of self and leads to overwhelming doubt about her maternal ability (Bennett, Boon, Romans, & Grootendorst, 2007).

Beck interviewed various women who have recovered from of postpartum illness and used identified themes from these interviews to categorize perinatal depression in four general stages. During the first stage, titled "encountering terror," a mother may feel consumed with overwhelming anxiety, terror, irrational irritability, and fears about her infant's welfare. During this stage, mothers may struggle with obsessive or intrusive thoughts and/or images that prey on their fear that "something bad will happen" to the infant, which would then validate their fear that they "failed" in their role as mother (Beck, 2006; Robertson et al., 2003). Other symptoms that contribute to a mothers feeling despair include irrational emotions, inability to function, invasive thought, pervasive anxiety, and social withdrawal (Bennett et al., 2007). Irrational emotions are often manifested in episodes of sadness, anxiety, irritability, anger, crying and worrying (Bennett et al., 2007).

Beck's second stage of perinatal depression is "dying of self" (Beck, 2006) and addresses the fact that many depressed mothers felt like they were a "different person"; the essence of who they were prior to parenthood had disappeared. During this stage, women described feeling of a loss-of-control and a sense of individual loss (Robertson et al., 2003). In this stage, women had difficulty reaching out to others, which often led to the loss of relationships. Depressed mothers struggled with multiple areas of impaired performance ranging from simple activities like personal hygiene to a more complex tasks like working inside/outside the home (Bennett et al., 2007).

Beck's third stage of perinatal depression is "*struggling to survive.*" In this stage, a mother may actively attempt to reach out for support from family members, health care workers or individuals within religious organizations (Beck, 2006). Sometimes, these mothers become more distressed as they feel their concerns about their depressed state may have been ignored or minimized by health care provider and/or family member, which led to mothers feeling disappointed, frustrated, humiliated and angry (Robertson et al., 2003).

Beck's final stage of perinatal depression is "regaining control" (Beck, 2006). The majority of mothers with perinatal depression can and do recover from depression Once she is in recovery, a mother may see preceding months as an empty memory, resulting in them feeling "robbed" of time to bond with their infant (Beck, 2006). A mother may grieve over this "lost time" and fear that this lost time will lead to permanent bonding problems and irreversibly lead to negative consequences for her infant.

Perinatal Anxiety Disorders

> "I was anxious all the time. What if something happened to her? What if she stopped breathing? What if she kept crying and I wasn't able to soothe her?"
>
> "Having worked in health care, I couldn't stop ruminating on the 'what if.' I took care of other people's kids all day and have seen them go downhill fast. I couldn't stop worrying about something happening to my child. Every time I took care of a sick child, I imagined such illness happening to my daughter."
>
> (Anonymous active duty military parent/patient)

Generalized anxiety disorder occurs in 1.3%–8.5% of women during pregnancy and 4.4%–8.2% of women between birth and 3 months postpartum (Williams, 2014). Most often, the focus of a pregnant woman's anxiety centers around pregnancy-related fears and worries (Brunton, Dryer, Saliba, & Kohlhoff, 2015). Perinatal anxiety is more prevalent in the antenatal period compared to postpartum period, whereas perinatal depression is more frequent in the postpartum period. The presence of antepartum anxiety creates *threefold* increased risk of developing subsequent postpartum depression (Williams, 2014).

Perinatal anxiety negatively affects the developing baby due to the influence of mothers' HPA stress hormone axis on her developing infant (Somerville et al., 2014). The effect of perinatal anxiety on the developing fetus will be discussed in subsequent chapters.

In addition to the effect of anxiety on developing infant, pregnant women with anxiety frequently are more distressed about physical changes in pregnancy, take more sick leave during pregnancy, make more visits to an obstetrician, and have increased likelihood of developing fear of childbirth that may result in a woman requesting an elective cesarean section (Rubertson, Hellstrom, Cross, & Sydsjo, 2014).

Perinatal Obsessive-Compulsive Disorder

> "When he cried, I tried to think of ways to get him to stop. I thought of smothering him with a pillow. What was I thinking? I would snap out of that thought, reassure myself that I could never do such a thing, and go on. These were just random disturbing ideas. Still, I hadn't thought about such things before."
>
> (An anonymous patient)

Obsessive-Compulsive Disorder (OCD) was previously classified as an anxiety disorder in DSM-IV, but is now in its own separate category in DSM-5 (American Psychiatric Association [APA], 2013). Obsessions are recurrent or persistent thoughts, urges or images that are experienced as intrusive and unwanted and cause marked anxiety or distress (APA, 2013). Compulsions are repetitive behaviors that an individual feels driven to perform in response to obsessive/intrusive thoughts and not a realistic way of dealing with a situation (APA, 2013).

Perinatal OCD in pregnant and postpartum women occurs two times more often than in women in the general population (Stein, 2014). Recent studies have found Perinatal OCD rates ranging from 1.2% to 5.2% during pregnancy and 4% within 6 months postpartum (O'Hara et al., 2014; Williams, 2014). Antenatal OCD often presents with obsessions about fears of fetal death/contamination (Stein, 2014), while postpartum OCD may have obsessive thoughts about hurting their infant or worries about harm coming to their infant. Perinatal OCD obsessions, centered on the baby's welfare, are excessive in nature and can lead to compulsive and very frequent nighttime checking to ensure the safety of the child (Wisner, Peindl, Gigliotti, & Hanusa, 1999). Other times, obsessions manifest as intrusive thoughts that center on themes of contamination, causing harm to children, offensive violent/sexual images, religious preoccupations and urges for symmetry (Sit, Rothchild, & Wisner, 2006).

A frequent obsessive thought seen in perinatal OCD is a mother imagining that she will hurt her infant. To counter this obsessive thought, a mother may engage in compulsive checking behaviors or avoidance of objects/places that provoke anxiety (O'Hara et al., 2014). Women with perinatal OCD may very well develop comorbid anxiety and depressive disorder. One critical aspect of Perinatal OCD is differentiating obsessive thought from postpartum psychosis. Women with Perinatal OCD are greatly disturbed by their thoughts and hence rarely ever act on them (Sit et al., 2006). Given the intrusive thoughts, mothers may fear they are "going crazy" and that they are "bad mothers" and are frequently reluctant to disclose these thoughts to care providers due to the fear of the infant being taken away (O'Hara & McCabe, 2013).

Perinatal Posttraumatic Stress Disorder (PTSD)

> "I couldn't become attached to him because the last month of pregnancy I kept being told about the risk of labor. I had gone from a normal, healthy pregnancy to bed rest. I had to distance myself emotionally. I wasn't able to meet him immediately as he had to be taken to NICU. It was several days before I was able to see and hold my child. He didn't feel like mine. My Cesarean section scar serves as a reminder. Now, whenever I go to well checks, my heart rates increases, and I become anxious. I feel like I am a bad mother."
>
> (An anonymous patient partaking in a motherhood group)

Perinatal PTSD is based on the acknowledgment that birth can be a traumatic experience (Beck, Simkin, Storton, & Harrison, 2013; Reynolds, 1997). Perinatal PTSD occurs in approximately 2% of postpartum women (James, 2015). Of note, there are two main subdivisions of perinatal PTSD. One group of mothers experience perinatal PTSD secondary to a history of sexual trauma/abuse—the invasive procedures required for childbirth can thus trigger memories of past trauma (Grekin & O'Hara, 2014). In contrast, the other group subcategory of women with perinatal PTSD had perceived or experienced their childbirth experience as traumatic.

A perinatal PTSD diagnosis requires an individual to be exposed (exposed being defined as personally experienced or witnessed first hand) to a significant traumatic event that threatens bodily injury, death or sexual violence. In addition to exposure to the traumatic event, a woman must have symptoms in four categories of symptoms to include re-experiencing symptoms, avoidance, alterations in cognition and mood, as well as significant alterations in physiological arousal and reactivity (APA, 2013).

Re-experiencing symptoms are the most common PTSD symptoms seen in perinatal PTSD following traumatic childbirth (James, 2015). Re-experiencing symptoms can be seen as recurrent, involuntary and intrusive memories, recurrent or distressing dreams of dissociative reactions (flashbacks) wherein a mother feels like the trauma is recurring (APA, 2013). In some perinatal PTSD cases, women report flashbacks and distressing dreams related to their delivery experience. One clinical example is seen in a story shared by one mother who reported a traumatic experience where anesthesia wore off during her cesarean section, and she became cognizant during the cesarean—she regularly recalled the feeling of helplessness and horror. This mother would have recurring nightmares about her experience that led to challenges bonding with her child.

Avoidance is the second key feature in perinatal PTSD and seen an unconscious (or intentional) strategy to avoid re-experiencing the anxiety-provoking or distressing feelings related to her trauma. Women with perinatal PTSD try to avoid places/activities that will trigger trauma memories, avoid discussing any subject around the subject of labor or hospital; they withdraw from social activities with other moms. They may avoid interacting with their infant or be reluctant to engage in bonding activities. In more extreme cases, a mother may avoid taking her baby to well checks/receiving immunization because going to pediatrician/hospital triggers memories of trauma (James, 2015). Another key aspect of avoidance is the implication on a mother's health. Like PTSD due to other forms of trauma, avoidance frequently prevents a mother from disclosing her symptoms or seeking help. Often "seeking help" means she has to acknowledge she has a problem. Acknowledging this problem can precipitate painful memories and physical and psychological distress.

The third category of symptoms characteristic of PTSD includes negative alterations in cognition and mood (APA, 2013) this is seen as negative appraisal of one's trauma (James, 2015). Women with Perinatal PTSD develop negative appraisal of their birth experience as well as a struggle with automatic negative thoughts, flawed assumptions, and core beliefs about themselves and world around them (James, 2015). One example of this can be the mother who was determined to have a natural delivery but ended up requiring an emergency cesarean section. A mother in this situation may develop negative cognitions and feel that there is something wrong with her for not being able to deliver naturally. Women may also displace feelings and disappoint related to birth onto their infant and view her infant negatively because he or she was the cause of her of pain (James, 2015). The final category of symptoms includes changes in arousal or reactivity and can be seen as an irritable outburst, sleep disturbances, problems with concentration and self-destructive behavior. These symptoms frequently occur because the body is reacting to a memory of an event as it is a current threat (James, 2015).

One clinical example of Perinatal PTSD is as follows:

> A mother described her last pregnancy was otherwise routine until one day she presented for a well check after 30 weeks, and was told that, due to problems with the placenta, she was at high risk of miscarrying or having complicated delivery. Due to the nature of her obstetrical complication, she required delivery via caesarean via "classic" cesarean incision, which was more invasive than usual, and would result in larger scar down the center of the abdomen. Whenever this mother would look at her scar, she remembered her traumatic birth experience and period leading up to delivery. Whenever she went to the pediatrician for well child checks, her heart would start racing, she would get nervous and want to avoid the visit altogether.

Perinatal Bipolar Disorder

Perinatal bipolar disorder often initially presents similar to perinatal depression. While unipolar depression is thought to be primarily secondary to a deficiency in neurotransmitters, bipolar disorder is thought to be secondary to faulty excitatory/inhibitory pathways in parts of the brain responsible for emotion, impulse control and executive functioning (APA, 2013). In bipolar disorder, an individual has periods of depression, as well as a distinct period of opposite extreme called *mania*. Mania is characterized by oscillations in mood, energy and ability to function. When extreme energy is present, cognition and ability to access rational thought are compromised (APA, 2013; Chang, 2014). An individual's mood in mania is expansive and elevated and will likely vary with periods of irritability or extreme lability. These mood changes are accompanied by changes in cognition/perception that leads to poor decision-making and involvement in excessive activities that are often destructive or could result in painful consequences. An individual experiencing mania has decreased need for sleep and can feel rested from as little as 2 hours of sleep, or go several days without sleep and not need it. (Of note, in perinatal depression or anxiety disorders, a mother may have the inability to sleep or to adapt to a temporary role where one has less sleep—this is not the same as sleep changes seen in mania). The excessive energy in mania may be accompanied by racing, disconnected thoughts, and behaviors as well as pressured speech. While some individuals speak fast when nervous, a person with mania is nearly impossible to interrupt or redirect.

Milder versions of mania are called *hypomania* where symptoms are similar to mania, but milder in manner. Hypomania is manifested as an elevated mood, increased energy and distinct functional impairment. Because hypomania does not cause severe impairment and does not typically require hospitalization, it can be harder to recognize, diagnose and treat. Hypomania may present with increased productivity, creativity, as well as euphoria with minimal effect on occupational/social/emotional functioning. Due to euphoria, and increased productivity, individuals may be unwilling to seek or comply with treatment.

There are two subcategories of bipolar disorder classified as Bipolar I and Bipolar II. Bipolar I denotes mania, while Bipolar II denotes hypomania. Given the higher likelihood of a severe presentation, Bipolar I Disorder is much easier to detect than Bipolar II, and women with Bipolar I disorder have a 20–30% chance of developing postpartum psychosis (BeyondBlue, 2011).

Women with Bipolar I Disorder often struggle with severe functional impairment. One study found that 74% of mothers with Bipolar I may go on to develop postpartum psychosis (Sit et al., 2006). Frequent precipitants of postpartum bipolar disorder or postpartum psychosis include suddenly stopping mood stabilizer treatment due to concern about teratogenic effects of medication (Sit et al., 2006). In contrast, Bipolar II is more challenging to diagnosis as it frequently initially presents with depression, and hypomania symptoms are "sub-threshold" and usually predominantly manifest as depression.

Postpartum Psychosis

Postpartum psychosis is most frequently secondary to bipolar disorder and less often associated with a primary psychotic disorder such as schizophrenia. Bipolar disorder, particularly manic phase, presents with mood-congruent psychotic features. If there is significant mood component (euphoria or depression), then such is more suggestive of bipolar disorder with psychotic features than primary psychotic disorder (less common). Studies have found that 77%–88% of women with postpartum psychosis have bipolar or schizoaffective disorder compared with 12% having primary psychotic disorder (Paschetta et al., 2014). Finally, in less common cases, women with a history of unipolar depression can also have elevated risk of developing postpartum psychosis, as a major depressive disorder with mood-congruent psychotic features, even in the absence of bipolar illness (Mighton et al., 2015). A review of data by Mighton et al. examined the risks of postpartum psychosis in mothers with a history of unipolar depression (Mighton et al.,

2015). Mighton et al., found up to 23% of women with a history of unipolar depression went on to develop postpartum psychosis, but only experienced psychosis in the postpartum period (Mighton et al., 2015).

Postpartum psychosis occurs in 1–2 per 1,000 births and usually occurs within 2 weeks postpartum (Marder, 2014). Women are more likely to experience psychosis during postpartum period more so than any other time in their lives (Marder, 2014). By definition, psychosis is a disturbance in an individuals' perception of reality and is often exhibited through delusions (fixed false beliefs), hallucinations (false perceptions) and/or thought disorganization (Marder, 2014). Risk factors include the history of puerperal psychosis, history of bipolar disorder, family history of postpartum psychosis, first pregnancy or recent discontinuation of lithium or another mood stabilizer (Marder, 2014). Like the other perinatal mood and anxiety disorders, pathogenesis in the postpartum period is thought to be related to the effects of rapid hormone fluctuations on underlying bipolar disorder, as well as sleep deprivation (Marder, 2014). Women with psychosis may develop paranoia, grandiose/bizarre delusions, mood lability and perplexity (Paschetta et al., 2014; Sit et al., 2006). Postpartum psychosis may have relatively sudden onset of grossly disorganized behavior, poor insight and poor judgment that can have devastating consequences for both mother and offspring (Sit et al., 2006). Women with postpartum psychosis have unusual psychotic symptoms with mood-incongruent delusions of reference, persecution, jealousy and grandiosity as well as visual, tactile or olfactory hallucinations that usually are indicative of organic syndrome (Sit et al., 2006). Women with postpartum psychosis have 70-fold increased risk of suicide (Sit et al., 2006).

One of the most feared consequences of postpartum psychosis includes the development of homicidal thoughts that result in infanticide. Although approximately 28%–35% of women hospitalized with postpartum psychosis endorse delusions about their infant, only 9% of these women had thoughts of harming their infant (Sit et al., 2006). Given severe consequences of postpartum psychosis to the mother and her child, it is considered an emergency that necessitates immediate evaluation or possible hospitalization (Sit et al., 2006).

Consequences of Perinatal Mood and Anxiety Disorders

To the Mother

Mood and anxiety disorders in the antepartum period are associated with premature births, intrauterine growth impairment, operative deliveries and admission to neonatal intensive care units (Thoppil, Riutcel, & Nalesnik, 2005). King et al. (2010) found the incidences of hyperemesis gravidarum, gestational diabetes, preeclampsia, obstetric cholestasis and placenta previa were positively correlated with prenatal anxiety and depression scores (King et al., 2010).

One of the most serious consequences of perinatal mood and anxiety disorders is the presence of suicidal ideations, suicide attempts or deaths by suicide. Over 90% of individuals who die by suicide have a diagnosable mood disorder at the time of suicide (Gentile, 2011).

Suicidal thoughts and suicidal ideations increase the likelihood of suicide attempts and deaths by suicide. In the Western world, epidemiological researchers have demonstrated suicidal ideations occur in 13.1% to 33% of pregnant women (Gentile, 2011). Other studies have found that up to half of pregnant women referred for psychiatric care already have a history of self-harm, yet only 20% of women with suicidal thoughts share information with health care provider. Untreated perinatal mood disorder have higher incidence of suicidality in the perinatal period (Kim et al., 2015). Risk factors that contribute to suicidal behaviors include intimate partner violence, unmarried status, pregnancy outside of marriage, poor social support (Gentile, 2011). When pregnant women attempt suicide, the most frequent methods include poison ingestion or overdose, with the highest risk in the second trimester (Gentile, 2011). Despite evidence of high suicide attempts, the deaths by suicide are low (Gentile, 2011).

In contrast to the antenatal period, in the postpartum period, suicide is a leading cause of death with a least two new mothers out of 1,000 suffering from depression with suicidal tendencies (Pope, Sharma, & Campbell, 2013). Of these women with suicidal tendencies, 20%–30% will attempt suicide (Pope et al., 2013). Women with postpartum depression, postpartum bipolar disorder and postpartum psychosis are at increased risk of attempting suicide. In particular, women who were vulnerable to psychiatric illness during pregnancy have a risk for relapse, which subsequently increases the likelihood of suicide (Pope et al., 2013) with 70 times greater risk in the first year postpartum (Gentile, 2011). When a woman dies by suicide, her death has an extensive impact on her infant, her family and community. At times, maternal suicide is combined with a murder-suicide, as a mother will often kill her child and herself.

One example of attempted murder-suicide was seen in March of 2013 when national headlines told the story of Cynthia Wachenheim, a lawyer on postpartum maternity leave, killed herself and almost killed her child. (Hartocollis & Ruderman, 2013).

Mrs. Wachenheim left a suicide note in which she described how her 8-month-old son had tumbled twice. Wachenheim described these "two shameful incidents," wherein her son fell from a Gymini play set onto the wood floor when she walked out of the room for 5 minutes, and another time, her son fell off a bed. Mrs. Wachenheim felt ashamed and felt he had a concussion from these incidents that would harm him for the rest of his life (Hartocollis & Ruderman, 2013). Despite reassurance from her husband and pediatrician, Mrs. Wachenheim believed her son exhibited signs of illness that only a mother could see. She decided that she could not bear the thought of him suffering the rest of his life because of her actions, so she strapped him in a baby carrier on her and jumped out of an eight-story window, falling to her death (Hartocollis & Ruderman, 2013). Although she died instantly upon hitting the ground, miraculously, she ended up breaking her son's fall, and he bounced off her and only suffered a bruised cheek (Hartocollis & Ruderman, 2013). Mrs. Wachenheim's story grabbed national attention and focused it on postpartum depression. Most maternal suicides do not make the headlines, and consequently the family members suffer in silence.

To the Infant

One of the most significant consequences of maternal depression are the implications for the infants and mother–infant dyad. Perinatal depression causes adverse effects to mother–infant relationship. As previously mentioned, maternal depression predisposes mothers to less likelihood of engaging in childhood safety and preventive checks which are essential for infant's physical well-being (Grace, & Sansom, 2003). The impact of maternal mental health and the impact on the infant's mental health will be explored in the next chapter.

The Marriage and Social Relationships

In addition to risks to the mother, postpartum depression often leads to difficulties with interpersonal relationships to include social relationships, marital relationships, mother–child relationships, as well as negative consequences overall to the family unit (Earls, 2010). Research has also shown that maternal depression affects a women's perception of the quality of her intimate relationships and social supports. In particular, postpartum depression has been associated with increased rates of marital conflict, separation and divorce, which can then exacerbate maternal depression (Earls, 2010; Mulcahy, Reay, & Wilkinson, 2010). Maternal depression often leads to relationship distress such as fear of rejection from a partner, misdirected anger, withdrawal, marital dissatisfaction, as well as difficulties communicating needs.

Partners and family members may feel pushed away from the struggling mother and "left in dark" about the mother's turmoil, not understanding why the new mother cannot seem to be happy about her new role (Goodman & Santangelo, 2011).

Summary

The goal of this chapter is to increase awareness about the various causes of perinatal mood and anxiety disorders. We hoped to review various mood and anxiety disorders that occur in pregnancy and the perinatal period with a desire to increase awareness (Russell, Lang, Clinton, Adams, & Lamb, 2013) and to describe the impact of these disorders on women and communities.

In the following chapters, we will discuss infant mental health and perinatal mental health in fathers.

References

American Academy of Pediatrics. (2011). *Policy Statement: Screening for Postpartum Depression at Well-Child Visits.* LA Best Babies Network. (Accessed December 2015). Retrieved from https://laperinatalmentalhealth.files.wordpress.com/2010/06/screeening-at-well-child-visits.pdf

American Psychiatric Association. (Ed.) (2013). *DSM-5 Criteria: American Psychiatric Association.* Arlington, VA: Author.

Beck, C. T. (2006). Postpartum depression: It isn't just the blues. *American Journal of Nursing, 106*(5), 40–50.

Beck, C., Simkin, P., Storton, S. & Harrison, P. (2013, June). *PTSD, Birth Trauma, and Perinatal Mental Health.* Presented at Postpartum Support International 26th Annual Conference: Innovation and Advocacy to Support the Mental Health of Pregnant and Postpartum Families, Minneapolis, MN.

Bennett, H., Boon, H., Romans, S., & Grootendorst, P. (2007). Becoming the best mom that I can: Women's experiences of managing depression during pregnancy—a qualitative study. *BMC Women's Health,* 7(13). Retrieved from http://bmcwomenshealth.biomedcentral.com/articles/10.1186/1472-6874-7-13

BeyondBlue. (2011). Clinical Practice Guidelines: Depression and Related Disorders-Anxiety, Bipolar Disorder and Puerperal Psychosis—in the Perinatal Period—A Guidelines for Primary Care Health Professionals: Australian Government: National Health and Medical Research Counsel. Retrieved from www.beyondblue.org.au

Brunton, R., Dryer, R., Saliba, A., & Kohlhoff, J. (2015). Pregnancy anxiety: A systematic review of current scales. *Journal of Affective Disorders, 176,* 24–34.

Chang, K. (2014). *Bipolar and Related Disorders American Psychiatric Publishing Textbook of Psychiatry.* Washington, DC: American Psychiatric Association.

Downs, D., DiNallo, J., & Kirner, T. (2008). Determinants of pregnancy and postpartum depression: Prosepective influences of depressive symptoms, body image satisfaction, and exercise behavior. *Annuals of Behavioral Medicine, 36,* 54–63.

Earls, M. F., (2010). Committee on Psychosocial Aspects of Child & Family Health, American Academy of Pediatrics. Incorporating recognition and management of perinatal and postpartum depression into pediatric practice. *Pediatrics, 126*(5), 1032–1039. doi: 10.1542/peds.2010-2348

Gentile, S. (2011). Suicidal mothers. *Journal of Injury and Violence Research, 3*(2), 90–97.

Goodman, J., & Santangelo, G. (2011). Group treatment for postpartum depression: A systematic review. *Archives of Women's Mental Health, 14,* 277–293. doi:10.1007/s00737-011-0225-3

Gow, R., Lydecker, J., Lamanna, J., & Mazzeo, S. (2012). Representations of celebrities' weight and shape during pregnancy and postpartum: A Content analysis of three entertainment magazine websites. *Body Image, 9,* 172–175.

Grace, S., & Sansom, S. (2003). The effect of postpartum depression on the mother-infant relationships and child growth and development. In D. Stewart, E. Robertson, C. Dennis, S. Grace, & T. Wallington (Eds.), *Postpartum Depression: Literature Review of Risk Factors and Interventions.* University Health Network Women's Health Program. World

Health Organization. Retrieved from http://www.who.int/mental_health/prevention/suicide/lit_review_postpartum_depression.pdf

Grekin, R., & O'Hara, M. (2014). Prevalence and risk fctors of postpartum posttraumatic stress disorder: A meta-analysis. *Clinical Psychology Review, 34*, 389–401.

Hartocollis, A., & Ruderman, W. (2013). Mother called her final act evil. *The New York Times*. March 14, 2013. Retrieved from www.nytimes.com

Indman, P., Meyer, B., & Davis, W. (2013). *Perinatal Mood and Anxiety Disorders: Components of Care: Postpartum Support International (PSI) Pre-Conference Certificate Training*. Presented 2 days prior to 26th Annual Conference: Innovation and Advocacy to Support the Mental Health of Pregnant and Postpartum Families, Minneapolis, MN.

James, S. (2015). Women's experiences of symptoms of Posttraumatic Stress Disorder (PTSD) after traumatic childbirth: A review and critical apprasial. *Archives of Women's Mental Health*. Retrieved from https://www.ncbi.nlm.nih.gov/pmc/articles/PMC4624822/pdf/737_2015_Article_560.pdf

Kim, J., Porte, L., Saleh, M., Allweiss, S., Adams, M., Zhou, Y., & Silver, R. (2015). Suicide risk among perinatal women who report thoughts of self harm on depression screens. *Obstetrics & Gynecology, 125*(4, April), 885–893.

Kimmel, M., Hess, E., Roy, P., Palmer, J., Meltzer-Brody, S., Meuchel, J., . . . Payne, J. (2015). Family history, not lack of medication use, is associated with the development of postpartum depression in a high-risk sample. *Archives of Women's Mental Health, 18*, 113–121.

King, N. M. A., Chambers, J., O'Donnell, K., Jayaweera, S. R., Williamson, C., & Glover, V. A. (2010). Anxiety, depression and saliva cortisol in women with a medical disorder during pregnancy. *Archives of Women's Mental Health, 13*, 339–345.

Lawson, A., Murphy, K., Sloan, E., Uleryk, E., & Dalfen, A. (2015). The relationship between sleep and postpartum mental disorders: A systematic review. *Journal of Affective Disorders, 176*, 65–77.

Maia, B. R., Pereira, A. T., Marques, M., Bos, S., Soares, M. J., Valente, J., . . . Macedo, A. (2012). The role of perfectionism in postpartum depression and symptomatology. *Archives Women's Ment Health, 15*, 459–468. doi:10.1007/s00737-012-0310-2

Mighton, C., Inglis, A., Carrious, P., Hippman, C., Morris, E., Andrighetti, H., . . . Austin, J. (2015). Perinatal psychosis in mothers with a history of major depressive disorder. *Archives of Women's Mental Health, 19*(2), 253–258.

Mulcahy, R., Reay, R., & Wilkinson, R. (2010). A randomized control trial for the effectiveness of group interpersonal psychotherapy for postnatal depression. *Archives of Women's Mental Health, 13*(2), 125–139.

National Institute of Health and Care Excellence (NICE). (2014). Antenatal and postnatal mental health: Clinical Management and service guidelines. *Clinical Guideline*, December 17, 2014. Retrieved from www.Nice.org.uk/guidance/cg192

Newport, J., Fernandez, B. A., Juric, S., & Stowe, Z. (2014). Chapter 64: Psychopharmacology During Pregnancy and Lactation. In A. Schatzberg & C. Nemeroff (Eds.), The American psychiatric publishing textbook of psychopharmacology (4th ed.). Arlington, VA: American Psychiatric Publishing.

O'Hara, M., & McCabe, J. (2013). Postpartum depression: Current status and future directions. *Annual Review of Clinical Psychology, 9*, 379–407.

O'Hara, M., Wisner, K., Asher, N., & Asher, H. (2014). Perinatal mental illness: Definition, description and aetiology. *Best Practice & Research Clinical Obstetrics and Gynecology, 28*, 3–12.

Paris, R., Bolton, R. E., & Weinberg, M. K. (2009). Postpartum depression, suicidality, and mother-infant interactions. *Archives Women's Mental Health, 12*, 309–321. doi:10.1007/s00737-009-0105-2

Paschetta, E., Berrisford, G., Coccia, F., Whitmore, J., Wood, A., Sam, P., & Ismail, K. P. (2014). Perinatal psychiatric disorders: An overview. *American Journal of Obstetrics and Gynecology, 210*(6), 501–509.

Payne, J. (2016). *Postpartum Psychosis: Epidemiology, Clinical Manifestations, Assessment and Diagnosis*. In: Marder, S. (Ed.) UpToDate, Post TW, UpToDate, Waltham, MA. http://www.uptodate.com/contents/postpartum-psychosis-epidemiology-clinical-manifestations-assessment-and-diagnosis

Polak, M., Houghton, L., Reeder, A., Harper, M., & Conner, T. (2014). Serum 25-hyrdoxy vitamin D concentrations and depressive symptoms among young adult men and women. *Nutrients, 6*, 4720–4730.

Pope, C., Sharma, V., & Campbell, K. (2013). A prospective study of thoughts of self-harm and suicidal ideation during the postpartum period in women with mood disorders. *Archives of Women's Mental Health, 16*, 483–488.

Rechenberg, K., & Humphries, D. (2013). Nutritional interventions in depression and perinatal depression. *Yale Journal of Biology and Medicine, 86*, 127–137.

Reynolds, J. (1997). Post-traumatic stress disorder after childbirth: The phenomenon of traumatic birth. *Canadian Medical Association Journal, 156*(6), 831–835.

Robertson, E., Celasun, N., & Stewart, D. (2003). Risk factors for postpartum depression. In D. Stewart, E. Robertson, C. Dennis, S. Grace, & T. Wallington, (Eds.), *Postpartum Depression: Literature Review of Risk Factors and Interventions*. University Health Network Women's Health Program.

Robinson, M., Whitehouse, A., Newnham, J., Gorman, S., Jacoby, P., Holt, B., . . . Kusel, M. (2014). Low maternal serum vitamin D during pregnancy and the risk for postpartum depression symptoms. *Archives of Women's Mental Health, 17*, 213–219.

Rubertson, C., Hellstrom, J., Cross, M., & Sydsjo, G. (2014). Anxiety in early pregnancy; prevalence and contributing factors. *Archives of Women's Mental Health, 17*, 221–228.

Russell, S., Lang, B., Clinton, J., Adams, C., & Lamb, J. (2013). Perinatal mental health experiences of women and health professionals. *Boots Family Trust Alliance*. Retrieved from https://www.tommys.org/sites/default/files/Perinatal_Mental_Health_Experiences%20of%20women.pdf

Sit, D., Rothchild, A., & Wisner, K. (2006). A review of postpartum psychosis. *Journal of Women's Health, 15*(4), 352–368.

Sloan, E. (2011). Sleep deprivation and postpartum mental health case report. *Archives Women's Mental Health, 14*, 509–511. doi:10.1007/s00737-011-0247-x

Somerville, S., Dedman, K., Hagan, R., Oxnam, E., Wettinger, M., Byrne, S., . . . Page, A. (2014). The perinatal anxiety screening scale: Developmental and preliminary validation. *Archives of Women's Mental Health, 17*(5), 443–454.

Stein, M. (2014). *Obsessive-Compulsive Disorder in Pregnant and Postpartum Women*. In: UpToDate, Post TW (Ed.), UpToDate, Waltham, MA. (Accessed on June, 2015.) http://www.uptodate.com/contents/obsessive-compulsive-disorder-in-pregnant-and-postpartum-women

Thoppil, J., Riutcel, T., & Nalesnik, S. (2005). Early intervention for perinatal depression. *American Journal of Obstetrics and Gynecology, 192*, 1446–1448.

Verinder, S., & Mazmanian, D. (2003). Sleep loss and postpartum psychosis. *Bipolar Disorders, 5*, 98–105.

Ward-Zimmerman, B., & Verdetti, J. (2014). Addressing maternal mental health in the pediatric medical home. *IMPACT, Child Health and Development Institute of Connecticut.* Retrieved from www.chdi.org

Williams, J. (2014). Best practice guidelines for mental health disorders in the perinatal period. *BC Mental Health.* Retrieved from http://www.perinatalservicesbc.ca/health-professionals/guidelines-standards/maternal (Accessed on 24 January, 2016).

Wisner, K. L., Peindl, K. S., Gigliotti, T., & Hanusa, B. H. (1999). Obsessions and compulsions in women with postpartum depression. *Journal of Clinical Psychiatry, 60*(3), 176–180.

Yonkers, K., Wisner, K., Stewart, D., Oberlander, T., Dell, D., Stotland, N., . . . Lockwood, C. (2012). The management of depression during pregnancy: A report from the American Psychiatric Association and the American College of Obstetricians and Gynecologists. *FOCUS: The Journal of Lifelong Learning in Psychiatry, 10*(1), 78–89.

Chapter 3

Infant and Child Mental Health and Perinatal Illness

Melinda A. Thiam, Eric M. Flake, and Michael M. Dickman

What Is Infant Mental Health?

Infant mental health (IMH) addresses the emotional and social development of children from birth to 3 years of life. IMH expands the definition of an infant from 1 year (seen in primary care and pediatrics) to 3 years in order to recognize that the first 3 years of life are critical for overall infant development (Zeanah & Zeanah, 2009). In particular, IMH recognizes that early relationships will influence how a child learns to experience, tolerate and express a range of emotions, and form trusting relationships (Lieberman & Van Horn, 2008). The main concepts of infant mental health include acknowledgment that early interpersonal experiences matter and these experiences are carried out in the context of infant-caregiver relationship. The quality of these early relationships will influence developmental trajectories, thus negative relationships can impede development and precipitate future psychopathology (Zeanah & Zeanah, 2009). When psychopathology manifests early, intervention may help correct the negative developmental trajectories, while other times psychopathology that begins in infancy may be permanent.

Introduction to Infant Growth and Development

During the first 3 years of life, infants rapidly grow and develop across multiple domains (Rosenblum, Dayton, & Muzik, 2009). In just 36 months, infants will transition from completely helpless newborns, to complex creatures that can come and go as they please. Infants also learn that they can share thoughts, feelings and intentions with others, express themselves abstractly and empathize with others (Zeanah & Zeanah, 2009).

Physiological Development: It Starts In Utero!

During the early years of infancy, critical neuronal pathways are established by the stimulation infants receive from the environment, and these neuronal pathways develop as an infant responds to his or her environment (Baradon,

Broughton, Woodhead, & The Practice of Parent-Infant Project at the Anna Freud Center, 2005; Slade, Cohen, Sadler, & Miller, 2009). The infancy period has rapid neurological and physical development; for instance, at birth, an infant's brain is 25% of its adult weight, and by 2 years old, the infant's brain is 75% of adult weight (Baradon et al., 2005; Slade et al., 2009). Infant development begins in the prenatal environment and is influenced by maternal nutrition and maternal mental health (Baradon et al., 2005; Slade et al., 2009).

In pregnancy, maternal physiology has a significant and direct effect on fetal physiology. For instance, elevated stress hormones during pregnancy can negatively affect fetal physiology, which then predisposes the infant's neuroendocrine system to be hypo-reactive and less adaptable to stress (Davalos, Yadon, & Tregellas, 2012; Rifkin-Graboi, Borelli, & Enlow, 2009). Additionally, high maternal stress hormones lead to reduced uterine blood flow; which in turn can cause pregnancy complications such as low birthweight and/or prematurity (Goodman & Brand, 2009). High levels of fetal stress hormone can lead to negative effect on the infant's developing nervous system in areas of the brain that are critical to the development of memory as well as decreased reactivity of frontal lobe (Goodman & Brand, 2009; Kingston, McDonald, Austin, & Tough, 2015).

The birth process itself can also be potentially traumatic to infants (Baradon et al., 2005; Slade et al., 2009). At birth, infants have to adapt to rapid physiological changes as they leave the protective intrauterine environment and transition to a less regulated outside world. For example, notable changes in infant cardiovascular system require infants to shift from oxygenating through the placenta via mother's cardiovascular system and transition to using his or her own lungs for the first time. Disruptions in cardiopulmonary transition can lead to permanent birth defects. Immediately after birth, infants are now in cold, overstimulating environment that becomes their new world. Infants are bombarded by numerous external stimuli, strange sensations, while they are also introduced to the social world and are completely dependent on their parents for physical care essential for physical, social and emotional survival (Baradon et al., 2005; Slade et al., 2009). Fortunately, infants are biologically primed to seek out this infant–parent bond through programming to respond to their mother's voice (Chase-Brand, 2008). From this first "meeting" at birth, an infant and mother will continue to deepen their bond and relationship with one another, which will ensure the infant's physical survival as well as influence emotional and social development.

Infant Emotional Development

Infant emotional development directly correlates with changes in their physical development as well as cognitive and social functioning (Rosenblum et al., 2009). Key components of emotional development include learning how to relate to the outside world, regulating emotions, developing a sense of self, and reducing early anxiety (Baradon et al., 2005; Slade et al., 2009).

Emotional development begins in the first week of life as an infant starts to engage with his or her environment (Rosenblum et al., 2009). Newborn infants are capable of a limited range of discrete emotional expression; these expressions expand as they grow more responsive to their environment. A newborn's basic emotions include distressed negative emotions versus positive and stimulating emotions (Rosenblum et al., 2009). Distressed emotional expression is present at birth and will precipitate the development of discrete emotions such as sadness, disgust, fear, and anger (Rosenblum et al., 2009). Positive emotions (such as a smile) starts to emerge by 2–3 months of age; by 2 months old, infants are capable of recognizing faces and discriminating between distinct human expression and emotional intensity (Rosenblum et al., 2009). Although infants can detect emotions/emotional expression, they are not able to understand these emotions and are fully dependent on their caregiver and environment to help them interpret emotions. Infants learn to interpret and respond to emotion through the process of social referencing, which is how an infant uses other's expressions to help him or her know how to respond to the environment (Rosenblum et al., 2009). Infants also engage in social mirroring wherein they imitate facial expression of caregivers and use these interactions to help synchronize their expressions, gestures and vocalizations (Lieberman & Van Horn, 2008), which then facilitate the later development of empathy and mutuality (Lieberman & Van Horn, 2008).

For an infant to effectively learn how to effectively reflect his or her caregiver's interactions, a parent needs to be able to recognize his or her baby as a person with a mind and feelings and understand the infant's behaviors are a means to communicate these feelings (Baradon et al., 2005; Slade et al., 2009). Likewise, a parent must also be able to attune to his or her baby's emotional state. Attunement is the empathic responsiveness between two individuals where these individuals can share a specific emotion (Baradon et al., 2005; Slade et al., 2009). Attunement allows a parent to be mindful of his or her infants' nonverbal behaviors and help his or her infant moderate/interpret these emotions while also remaining separate. For example, a mother may demonstrate separateness from her infant by exaggerating her voice, widening her eyes, while also emphasizing that she registered his emotional state (Baradon et al., 2005; Slade et al., 2009).

When an infant interacts with his or her parents, these interactions follow meaningful patterns. When a mother responds to her infant's modified emotional state in a positive manner, her infant learns that his interactions have an impact on another and allow him to develop the ability to represent his thoughts/feelings through play and language (Baradon et al., 2005; Slade et al., 2009). The better a mother can interpret and respond to her child's intention, mood and affect, the faster the infant can develop the ability to represent his thoughts and feeling through language and play (Barlow & Svanberg, 2009). When the caregiver responds positively to his or her infant in this "mother–baby dance," and there is a synchronous relationship between the two, the infant learns self-regulation.

Self-regulation is critical to later development (Rosenblum et al., 2009) and allows an infant to learn how to respond to stress in the environment. When infants are exposed to extreme levels of environmental stress, they have reciprocal adaptive (or maladaptive) changes in multiple organ systems such as the developing brain, neuroendocrine system, immune system, metabolic system and cardiovascular system (Baradon et al., 2005).

Infant Social Development

Social development begins with the parent-infant relationship, and to a lesser extent, other relationships such as peers, extended family and childcare relationships (Rosenblum et al., 2009). Key components of social development include the formation of an attachment, the development of infant-parent dyad, the establishment of a sense of self and transition from separation to individuation (Baradon et al., 2005; Slade et al., 2009).

Attachment is a special and powerful relationship that develops between an infant and his or her caregiver during the first year of life (Baradon et al., 2005; Slade et al., 2009). An infant's ability to securely relate to his or her primary caregiver (traditionally the mother) will form the basis of attachment (Simpson et al., 2015) and will influence all other aspects of infant development (Baradon et al., 2005; Slade et al., 2009). A positive attachment is essential in establishing the child's sense of safety and security, influences the infant's fundamental modes of regulating his thoughts and feelings, and influences the quality of his capacity to explore the world productively and autonomously (Baradon et al., 2005; Slade et al., 2009).

The caregiver–infant relationship forms the foundation of how an infant learns how to interact with others and serves to assist an infant in regulating his or her affect and learning to regulate arousal (Rosenblum et al., 2009). Infants with secure attachment become individuals who grow up to be sensitive and responsive to others and have a solid foundation for emotional regulation, self-esteem, and social adeptness (Baram, Davis, Obenaus, Sandman, & Small, 2012).

To foster an attachment relationship, infants intently monitor the emotional state and nonverbal communications of their mother and modify their behavior (Barlow & Svanberg, 2009; Rosenblum et al., 2009). Infants are motivated to maintain and preserve their relationship with their primary caregiver, and they will adapt their behavior to achieve this goal of preserving this relationship (Araneda et al., 2010). When an infant observes a negative response from his or her caregiver, he or she unconsciously adapts his or her behavior to elicit a rewarding response from his or her mother. Behaviors, feelings and thoughts that would elicit negative reaction are then excluded from consciousness and split off from self-experience (Barlow & Svanberg, 2009; Rosenblum et al., 2009).

Early Experience Matters: Foundations of the Caregiving Relationship

The development of the parent–infant dyad is critical in the formation of attachment and subsequent social-emotional development (Rosenblum et al., 2009). Traditionally, the dyadic relationship was assumed to be just mother–infant. Today, with recognition of the fatherhood role, there is greater emphasis on the triadic relationship, that is, both parents and their interactions with the infant. The psychology of fatherhood and father–infant interactions will be explored in a subsequent chapter, so for simplicity, the remainder of this chapter will refer to mother–infant dyad (Baradon et al., 2005; Slade et al., 2009).

Contributions of Infant to Dyad

An infant's health, developmental progression, and temperament can all affect the mother–infant relationship and subsequent attachment relationship (Baradon et al., 2005; Slade et al., 2009). For example, infants in Neonatal Intensive Care Unit (NICU) have higher levels of distress compared to infants of healthy parents (Yurdakul et al., 2009) and often have delayed bonding due to physical separation from their parent (Yurdakul et al., 2009). Additionally, infants treated in the NICU are usually premature and frequently have more cognitive, behavioral, socio-emotional and school problems when compared with control children, even in the absence of major neurosensory or motor impairments (Forcada-Guex, Pierrehumbert, Borghini, Moessinger, & Muller-Nix, 2006). Children with genetic syndromes, special needs or developmental delays also are at risk of developing unhealthy attachment relationships.

All healthy newborns show varying states of reactivity that describes infant arousal and emotion—these states include initial regulation orientation to visual stimuli, irritability and activity, soothability and overall susceptibility to distress (Rothbart, 2011). The intensity of these states vary from child to child and will be reflected in an infant's emotional and physiological current presentation and regulation (Rothbart, 2011). A child's reactive distress to particular stimuli occurs in the context of caregiver's soothing (Rothbart, 2011). For example, inconsolable and prolonged crying (> 20min per day) leads to parental frustration that subsequently leads to higher parental stress, lower parenting confidence, and causes a mother to perceive that she is unable to soothe her infant (Radesky et al., 2013). Infant crying can then lead to the occurrence of intrusive and hostile thoughts toward one's infant (Fairbrother, Barr, Pauwels, Brant, & Green, 2015).

Infant temperament (or more appropriately "perception" of temperament) influences parental actions in daily caregiving activities (Mantymaa,

Puura, Luoma, Salmalin, & Tamminen, 2006). Infants who are perceived as more difficult may receive less responsive mothering (Mantymaa et al., 2006; Rothbart, 2011), while parents respond with greater sensitivity to infants that are perceived as more soothable (Rothbart, 2011). While infant temperament is important in influencing the infant–parent relationship, the mother's perception of her infant's temperament is more influential in affecting mother–child relationship. Mental health or emotional distress in caregivers can negatively distort parental perception of the child (Mantymaa et al., 2006), and depressed mothers frequently perceive their infants as more problematic than healthy mothers (Mantymaa et al., 2006).

Contributions of Parent to Dyad

Parenting is an approximate process, and there is no such thing as the "perfect parent" (Baradon et al., 2005; Slade et al., 2009). Instead, psychology literature emphasizes that parents do not need to be perfect, but "good enough" (Baradon et al., 2005; Slade et al., 2009). "Good enough mothering" is achieved through a mother's capacity to tolerate developmental states of her baby, attune to her baby's needs, see her baby as a human person with feelings and intentions, and be able to respond contingently to her baby's communication (Baradon et al., 2005; Slade et al., 2009). A "good enough" mother is capable of accepting mismatches between her fantasies/expectations, accept the reality of her infant's individual characteristics, and will modify her behavior to provide the kind of care needed for her child (Lieberman & Van Horn, 2008).

Perception/Acceptance of Pregnancy

Establishing an emotional connection to the fetus is an important part of identifying with the maternal role (McFarland et al., 2011). During pregnancy, attachment to the fetus may be demonstrated through thoughts and feeling towards her unborn baby, as well as intentional beneficial changes in lifestyle for the sake of her infant (McFarland et al., 2011). Unwanted pregnancy and undesired timing can have a significant impact on prenatal attachment (Lederman & Weis, 2009).

Parent Behaviors: Sensitivity and Responsiveness

Maternal sensitivity is defined as a mother's ability to perceive her infant's signals accurately, and respond appropriately (Baram et al., 2012). Maternal responsiveness is the degree a mother consistently responds to her infant's signals (Baram et al., 2012). Sensitive caregiving gives rise to secure attachment in infants, and secure attachment promotes optimal development (Wan & Green, 2009).

Maternal depression negatively affects maternal sensitivity and responsiveness. Maternal depression has been associated with reduced parenting responsiveness, affection, increased intrusion and punitiveness (Wan & Green, 2009). Depressed mothers also have low levels of positive affect, high levels of negative affect, and difficulties in regulating emotions and behavior (Goodman & Brand, 2009). Compared to mothers without depression, depressed mothers differ from the way they perceive infant emotion and the way they respond to infant utterances as well as positive/negative infant facial expressions (Goodman & Brand, 2009; Hart, Field, & Roitfarb, 1999). Depressed mothers may respond to their infant with avoidant/withdrawn responses, or respond with hostile-intrusive overstimulation (Carnegie et al., 2015; Goodman & Brand, 2009). For example, mothers with depression are observed to be more physically intrusive and interfering with infant's exploratory activities (Field et al., 2001).

Past Experiences

Past experiences of trauma and loss can impact parenting. Mothers who are survivors of childhood sexual/emotional abuse may have a harder time adapting to parenting (Muzik et al., 2013). During observed mother–child interaction, mothers with childhood sexual abuse histories are more likely to be emotionally withdrawn or permissive in their parenting or more frequently exhibit hostile parenting (Muzik et al., 2013). Women with past abuse histories may also express more negative views of themselves as parents, have a less balanced perception of parenting, and show distorted representations toward parenting (Muzik et al., 2013). Adverse childhood experience often leads to the intergenerational *transmission of trauma*; a term that describes concept that unresolved psychological conflict from mother's childhood will affect her ability to interact with her infant (Lieberman & Van Horn, 2008). A mother's attachment history can impact the dyadic relationship with her infant. It has been hypothesized that a mother with poor attachment is at elevated risk of depression as well as impaired mother–infant bonding (Baram, et al., 2012).

Consequences of Negative Infant Mental Health

> "I think back to the early days of my daughter's life. For several months, I had suffered from depression, but I didn't realize how much it was affecting me. Now I feel like a horrible mother. . . . I missed out on several months of my daughter's life. I feel like a horrible mother—what kind of mother does this?"

Stress can affect an infant's development when the intensity of frightening events becomes unmanageable to an infant to the point of threatening physical and psychological integrity (Lieberman & Van Horn, 2008). One of the core damages, when this infant psychopathology occurs, is disrupted development (Lieberman & Van Horn, 2008).

Physical Consequences

When a mother is depressed, she becomes more sensitive to stress, which in turn leads to poor stress tolerance, cognitive distortion and negative influence on her physical ability to protect and care for the physical needs of her infant (Lieberman & Van Horn, 2008). Consequences of depression can lead to a mother not being able to read basic signals such as an indication of hunger or physical distress. Depressed mothers often have less healthy feeding and sleep practices for their infants, which can increase the likelihood of infant's undernourishment/stunted growth (Chase-Brand, 2008). Depressed mothers are less likely to engage in health practices such as keeping up to date with immunizations and increased likelihood of missing well-baby appointments, yet are more likely to have emergency room visits and less likely to engage in safety precautions such as using car seats, safety latches, and childproofing their home (Chase-Brand, 2008).

Infants of depressed mothers can also develop infant depression. One of the first manifestations of infant depression in developed countries is a non-organic failure to thrive (Guedeney, 1997). Non-organic failure to thrive (NOFTT) is a pediatric classification that describes infant depression (Chase-Brand, 2008). During the process of becoming depressed, an infant first starts to withdraw from social interaction followed by a display of more negative affect, less vocalization, and gaze aversion (Chase-Brand, 2008). These infants also vocalize less, mothers are less responsive to babies, and there is very little physical touch between infant and mother (Chase-Brand, 2008).

Mothers can be distressed to point they withdraw from their infant, or they become hostile and have increased the risk of physically harming their babies. Depressed mothers were more likely to use harsh punishment such as slapping an infant (Chase-Brand, 2008). Young children can be the victims of domestic violence; during the first year, more infants are abused than at any other one-year period (Lieberman & Van Horn, 2008). In severe maternal pathology, usually in the presence of psychotic symptoms, mothers experienced auditory hallucinations that could lead to child abuse and even, in rare cases, infanticide (Chase-Brand, 2008).

Effects on Social and Emotional Development

Poor attachment with caregivers and suboptimal emotional and social development can be enduring. Attachment theory is based on the four types of attachment patterns: secure attachment, anxious-avoidant, anxious-ambivalent, and disorganized attachment (Rosenblum et al., 2009). These basic attachment patterns were the result of the Strange Situation Protocol, wherein the interaction between a parent and a child is examined for separation and reunion (Rosenblum et al., 2009). In the secure attachment pattern, a parent left the room, the infant was distressed, but was able to be comforted/reassured upon the parent's return (Araneda, Santelices, & Farkas, 2010; Rosenblum et al., 2009). Anxious-ambivalent attachment occurs when a mother is not emotionally available to effectively attune to her infant, which leaves her infant with a sense of ambivalence and anxiety (Araneda et al., 2010). In anxious, avoidant attachment pattern, infants in the Strange Situation Protocol responded as if they did not need comfort from their parents. This observation was in conjunction with the observation that mother of these infants was frequently rejecting of infant distress. In turn, the mother's rejection of infant distress led to infants adapting their behavior to deactivate their emotional needs to preserve the relationship (Barlow & Svanberg, 2009; Rosenblum et al., 2009). Infants with avoidant attachment histories can then continue to struggle with subsequent relationships. They may expect rejection in relationships and are vulnerable to becoming insulted, hostile and potentially provoke adults/peers into rejecting them (Rosenblum et al., 2009).

In the anxious-ambivalent attachment, infants appeared desperate to have contact with their parents and were difficult to soothe upon reunion (Barlow & Svanberg, 2009; Rosenblum et al., 2009). Mothers of these infants were observed to be inconsistent with their care and most interactions with infants were not based off infant cues (Barlow & Svanberg, 2009; Rosenblum et al., 2009). Anxious-ambivalent infants were suspected to have heightened emotional activation with the goal to keep parents responsive and involved (Barlow & Svanberg, 2009; Rosenblum et al., 2009). Infants with ambivalent attachment learn to behave in an over-aroused manner in an attempt to receive emotional warmth that was offered inconsistently (Rosenblum et al., 2009). These individuals go on to be hesitant in exploring the novel situation, immature, easily frustrated, and less empathetic with their peers (Rosenblum et al., 2009).

In attachment theory, a mother's failure to respond to her infant's need for help can lead to an infant having difficulty in developing arousal modification (Goodman & Brand, 2009). Infants look to the mother for emotional attunement and regulation. During these interactions, an infant may become frustrated in attempts to obtain external regulation from his or her mother and subsequently turn to self-directed internal soothing behaviors when faced with stress (Goodman & Brand, 2009).

Another aspect of development impacted is an infant's emotional regulation and response to the environment. In response to their mother's effect, infants gaze less toward caregiver, are less playful, portray little positive effect and instead often appear emotionally withdrawn (Goodman & Brand, 2009; O'Hara & McCabe, 2013). Infants of depressed mothers are not as attuned to caregivers' verbal expression, are less playful and less interactive with their environment. When infants do not interact reciprocally with their caregiver, they may develop poor attachment. Poor attachment negatively affects social, cognitive and emotional growth and (Alhusen, Hayat, & Gross, 2013; Araneda et al., 2010; Erickson, 2013; Muzik et al., 2013; Rosenblum et al., 2009). One example of the effect of depressed mothers on infants was illustrated by the "still face procedure" where mothers were asked to engage in a period of face-to-face play, followed by a period where an adult holds a still face (restricted affect) and finally has re-engagement period with his or her infant (Erickson, 2013; Rosenblum et al., 2009). Normally, infants become distressed when they transition from interactive mirroring to still face phase because infants recognize that disruption in effective exchange is discrepant and undesirable (Rosenblum et al., 2009). In contrast, infants of depressed mothers reacted minimally when faced with the still face phase of the experiment (Erickson, 2013; Lavelli & Fogel, 2013; Stowe, 2012).

Effect on Long-Term Development

Consequences of child development extend beyond the first year. Without intervention, children whose mothers were depressed during first year show insecure attachments in toddlerhood and less interest in interacting with peers (Chase-Brand, 2008). Mothers with depression were less likely to talk or play with children and less likely to show their children books or keep their children on a daily routine (Chase-Brand, 2008). Due to less interaction, toddlers had diminished language skills and delayed cognitive development (Chase-Brand, 2008). Additionally, toddlers of depressed mothers demonstrate some problematic social and emotional issues. These include a decreased social competence, more internalizing, and externalizing behavior problems. Often, toddlers are more passive and withdrawn or more angry and aggressive. Preschool-age children of depressed mothers were viewed as more vulnerable and were at risk of lower cognitive scores (Bendell et al., 1994; Hay, 1997) and are at increased risk for developing extensive difficulties throughout childhood (Gladstone & Kaslow, 1994).

By middle childhood, children born to depressed mothers show less social competence and persistent disorganized attachment (Chase-Brand, 2008). They also may have increased the likelihood of school refusal, social anxiety, somatic complaints and depression (Chase-Brand, 2008). During the school-age years, children still require a secure parent–child attachment. From this attachment, they can learn life lessons regarding how to cope with stress, how to establish and maintain interpersonal relationships, how to regulate their emotions, and how to persist in the demands of daily life. Depressed parents often model ineffective coping responses and difficulties in their interpersonal relationships, which can result in a disorganized parent–child attachment.

Instead of the needed structure and routine, depressed parents provide a home environment that is more chaotic, less structured, less predictable and less nurturing than their non-depressed counterparts and frequently display ineffective and often harsh parental discipline technique. Parental responses may be erratic and inconsistent, vacillating between withdrawing from engaging with their children to responding in an explosive, volatile manner. These experiences contribute to the negative impact of maternal depression during the school-aged years.

School-age children of depressed parents also have shown higher levels of both externalizing and internalizing symptoms. They tend to be more prone to depression and anxiety, as well as less severe forms of emotional distress (Gladstone & Kaslow, 1994). School-age children of depressed mothers have higher rates of conduct disorder, ADHD, and other disruptive behavior disorders (Beardslee, Schultz & Selman, 1987) and tend to experience impaired academic performance, negative self-concept and negative self-esteem (Jaenicke et al., 1987). Children of depressed parents experience recurrent episodes of parent–child experiences of criticism, rejection, lack of warmth and intrusiveness develop a self–critical child with feelings of worthlessness that extend into adolescence (Koesterner, Zuroff, & Powers, 1991; Radye-Yarrow, Martinez, Mayfield, & Ronsaville, 1998).

Although the influence of parents' behavior is believed to diminish during the adolescent years, the cumulative effect of living with a parent who suffers from depression continues to impact into the teenage years. Many of the same aspects of the home environment, and parent–child relationship during the school-age years will continue into adolescence, with depressed parents being poor coping models, providing less monitoring and involvement with their child and utilizing damaging disciplining strategies. Critical developmental tasks during these years include the ability to develop a coherent sense of self, become less dependent upon the family, and establish meaningful, mature interpersonal relationships. These developmental tasks are difficult to achieve optimally within the context of a family with a depressed parent. A depressed parent who is having difficulty managing his/her personal stressors is not available to help the adolescent cope with the adolescent's set of stressful experiences.

While depressive disorders become more prevalent for adolescents themselves than earlier developmental stages, the youth of children depressed mothers are at an even higher risk of developing this disorder. When by parents with depression are raising adolescents, the strained family relationships often negatively influence peer relationships, lead to decreased school attendance, and academic problems. These adolescents are also reported to have an increased risk for substance abuse and a higher level of treatment for psychiatric disturbances. Most importantly, these youth are at higher risk for suicidal ideation and attempted/completed suicides.

Who Intervenes? Treating the Infant

Perinatal depression can have significant consequences if left untreated, and it is necessary for health care professionals to recognize treatment at all ages and take responsibility to assist the child and aid the depressed parent in obtaining treatment. The U.S. Preventive Services Task Force recommended that all adults in primary care be routinely screened for depression. Frequently, primary care clinics frequently use the PHQ-2 that asks a patient if they have felt down, depressed or hopeless as well as felt little interest or pleasure in doing things over the past 2 weeks. If the patient response is "yes," the provider should follow-up with additional questions and administer the PHQ (Olson, Dietrich, Prazar, & Hurley, 2006). In a similar fashion, infant mental health should also have involved provider screening for depression. Infant mental health is closely partnered and encompasses multiple disciplines. Most often, the provider completes an Infant Mental Health screening in pediatrics/family practice.

For new parents, the American Academy of Pediatrics has created a standard of 14 routine screenings during the IMH recognized "infancy" period (Simpson et al., 2015). Each of these routine screenings is a chance for assessment and intervention (Heneghan et al., 2007; Rafferty, Griffin, & Robokos, 2010). Pediatricians can be one of the key individuals to identify the problem and determine different means of intervention as they are often the only consistent health care contact encountered routinely by new mothers during first 2 years after giving birth (Liberto, 2012). Pediatricians and family medicine providers can assess the security of mother–infant bond as a means to detect potential maternal depression (Chase-Brand, 2008). Diminished eye contact, decreased smiling and reciprocal interactions may be present. A mother may also not attempt to soothe her crying infant and infant does not seem to calm into the mother's embrace (Chase-Brand, 2008). When an infant is showing signs of distress, addressing only the mother's depression is not sufficient. Other moderators that need to be taken into consideration for the child of a depressed parent would include age, sex, cognitive abilities (IQ), a healthy caregiver and sibling, the child's temperament, innate coping and social skills, as well as duration and severity of parental depression.

One simple technique to help with infant attachment and parental bonding that can be demonstrated in the provider's office is massage and skin to skin time. Massage and touch therapy is a simple, immediately implemented, and cost-effective method to strengthen an infant's sense of security. The intervention targeted at giving a sense of safety measured an infant's response to massage therapy versus a control group that was just rocked back and forth. After 6 weeks, infants in the massage group were felt to cry less and be more alert and interactive (Field, 1997).

To assist parents to become more engaged with their infant, additional coaching sessions modeling appropriate interaction and challenging mothers to maintain their baby's attentions may be required. Although pediatricians can refer mothers to their primary caregiver, in-home coaching and support is critical. Where available home visits help evaluate mother–infant relationship, therapists for mothers who are trained in perinatal mood and anxiety disorders may be able to perform mother–infant therapy in conjunction with therapy for the mother. These interventions have resulted in significant improvements in mother–infant interactions (Malphurs et al., 1996)

No single risk factor or child moderator stands alone in determining the outcome of children with a depressed parent. The cumulative results of the transactional nature–nurture interplay are what determine the end effects and functional ability of the child. Encouraging preventative family practices and responding appropriately to families with depressed parents is both possible and necessary for health care professionals caring for mothers and children. Additional screening interventions in primary care, as well as more treatment modalities, will be explored in a later part of this book.

Summary

Infant mental health is a wonderful example of how humans are interdependent on one another. Maternal depression does not exist in a vacuum. In one sense, infants are like the "canaries in a mine" to detect/give warning signs that something is going on with the mother. Although mothers may be less inclined to seek treatment, addressing infant mental health can engage the maternal instinct and does not "feel like" therapy treatment. A clinical example is a case of a mother who was struggling to admit that she was suffering from depression. Fortunately, this mother still sought help and was receiving treatment. As it so happened, this mother had family that was located far away. In a means to attempt to preserve family connection, she created video messages of herself and her daughter interacting together. One day, this mother was reviewing these video messages and had a moment of enlightenment. She noticed her nonverbal interactions with her infant and her infant's responsiveness significantly differed before and after treatment.

Given such an example, another possibility to help promote infant mental health is to encourage a mother or family member who is depressed to record themselves interacting with their infant. This process will allow a mother to see how she interacts with her infant and help her understand how maternal mental health is also infant mental health. In the next chapter, we will visit the other aspect of maternal mental health—that is paternal mental health.

References

Alhusen, J. L., Hayat, M. J., & Gross, D. (2013). A longitudinal study of maternal attachment and infant developmental outcomes. *Archives of Women's Mental Health, 16*, 521–529. doi:10.1007/s00737-013-0357-8

Araneda, M., Santelices, M., & Farkas, C. (2010). Building infant–mother attachment: The relationship between attachment style, socio-emotional well-being and maternal representation. *Journal of Reproductive and Infant Psychology, 28*(1), 30–43.

Baradon, T., Broughton, C., Woodhead, J., & P.-I. P. a. t. A. F. Centre. (2005). *The Practice of Psychoanalytic Parent-Infant Psychotherapy: Claiming the Baby.* New York, NY: Routledge.

Baram, T., Davis, E., Obenaus, A., Sandman, C., & Small, S. (2012). Fragmentation and unpredictability of early life experience in mental disorders. *American Journal of Psychiatry, 169*, 907–915.

Barlow, J., & Svanberg, P. (2009). *Keeping the baby in mind: Infant mental health in practice* [E-Reader Version]. New York: Routledge.

Beardslee, W., Schultz, L., & Selman, R. (1987). Level of social cognitive development, adaptive function and DSM-III diagnosis in adolescent offspring of parents with affective disorders: Implications of the development of the capacity for mutuality. *Developmental Psychology, 23*, 807–815.

Bendell, D., Field, T., Yando, R., Lang, C. Martinez, A., & Pickens, J. (1994). Depressed mothers' perception of their preschool children's vulnerability. *Child Psychiatry and Human Development, 24*, 183–190.

Carnegie, R., Shepherd, C., Pearson, R., Button, K., Munafo, M., Evans, J., & Penton-Voak, I. (2015). Changing mothers' perceptions of infant emotion: A pilot study. *Archives of Women's Mental Health, 19*, 167.

Chase-Brand, J. (2008). Effects of maternal postpartum depression on the infant and older siblings. In S. Stone & A. Menken (Eds.), *Perinatal and Postpartum Mood Disorders: Perspectives and Treatment Guide for the Health Care Practitioner.* New York: Springer.

Davalos, D., Yadon, C., & Tregellas, H. (2012). Untreated prenatal maternal depression and potential risk to offspring: A review. *Archives of Women's Mental Health, 15*, 1–14.

Erickson, M. (2013). *Supporting Secure Parent-Child Attachment in the Face of Maternal Depression and Other Risks.* Paper presented at the Postpartum Support Internation (PSI) 26th Annual Conference: Innovation and Advocacy to Support the Mental Health of Pregnant and Postpartum Families, Minneapolis, MN.

Fairbrother, N., Barr, R., Pauwels, J., Brant, R., & Green, J. (2015). Maternal thoughts of harm in response to infant crying: An experimental analysis. *Archives of Women's Mental Health, 18*, 447–455.

Field, T. (1997). The treatment of depressed mothers and their infants. In L. Murray & P. Cooper (Eds.), *Postpartum Depression and Child Development* (pp. 221–236). New York: Guilford Press.

Field, T., Diego, M., Dieter, J., Hernandez-Reif, M., Schanberg, S., Kuhn, C., . . . Bendell, D. (2001). Depressed, withdrawn and intrusive mother's effects on their fetuses and neonates. *Infant Behavior and Development, 24*, 27–39.

Forcada-Guex, M., Pierrehumbert, B., Borghini, A., Moessinger, A., & Muller-Nix, C. (2006). Early dyadic patterns of mother-infant interactions and outcomes of prematurity at 18 months. *Pediatrics, 118*, e107.

Gladstone, T. R. G., & Kaslow, N. J. (1994). Depression and attributions in children and adolescents: A meta-analytic review. *Journal of the American Academy of Child and Adolescent Psychiatry, 33*, 1265–1274.

Goodman, S., & Brand, S. (2009). Infants of depressed mothers: Vulnerabilities, risk factors, and protective factors for the later development of psychopathology. In C. Zeanah (Ed.), *Handbook of Infant Mental Health* (3rd ed., Ch. 9, pp. 153–170). New York, NY: The Guilford Press.

Guedeney, A. (1997). From early withdrawal reaction to infant depression: A baby alone does exist. *Infant Mental Health Journal, 18*(4), 339–349.

Hart, S., Field, T., & Roitfarb, M. (1999). Depressed mothers' assessment of their neonate's behaviors. *Infant Mental Health Journal, 20*(2), 200–210.

Hay, D. F. (1997). Postpartum depression and cognitive development. In L. Murray & P. J. Cooper (Eds.), *Postpartum Depression and Child Development* (pp. 85–110). New York: Guilford Press.

Heneghan, A. M., Chaudron, L., Storfer-Isser, A., Park, E. R., Kelleher, & K. J., Stein, R. (2007). Factors associated with the identification and management of maternal depression by pediatricians. *Pediatrics, 119*(3), 444–454.

Jaenicke, C., Hammen, C. L., Zupan, B., Hiroto, D., Gordon, D., Adrain, C., & Burge, D. (1987). Cognitive vulnerability in children at risk for depression. *Journal of Abnormal Child Psychology, 15*, 559–572.

Kingston, D., McDonald, S., Austin, M. P., & Tough, S. (2015). Association between prenatal and postnatal psychological distress and toddler cognitive development: A systematic review. *PLOS One*. Retrieved from http://journals.plos.org/plosone/article?id=10.1371/journal.pone.0126929.

Koesterner, R., Zuroff, D. C., & Powers, T. A. (1991). Family origins of adolescent self-criticism and its continuity into adulthood. *Journal of Abnormal Psychology, 100*, 191–197.

Lavelli, M., & Fogel, A. (2013). Interdyad differences in early mother–infant face-to-face communication: Real-time dynamics and developmental pathways. *Developmental Psychology, 49*(12), 2257–2271.

Lederman, R., & Weis, K. (2009). *Psychosocial Adaptation to Pregnancy: Assessment of Seven Dimensions of Maternal Role Development* (3rd ed.). New York: Springer.

Liberto, T. (2012). Screening for depression and help-seeking in postpartum women during well-baby pediatric visits: An integrated review. *Journal of Pediatric Health Care, 26*(2). doi:10.1016/j.pedhc.2010.06.012

Lieberman, A., & Van Horn, P. (2008). *Psychotherapy with Infants and Young Children: Repairing the Effects of Stress and Trauma on Early Attachment.* New York: The Guildford Press.

Malphurs, J. E., Field, T. M., Larranie, C., Pickens, J., Pelaez-Nogueras, M., Yondo, R., & Bendell, D. (1996). Altering withdrawn and intrusive interaction behaviors of depressed mothers. *Infant Mental Health Journal, 17*, 152–160.

Mantymaa, M., Puura, K., Luoma, I., Salmalin, R., & Tamminen, T. (2006). Mother's early perception of her infant's difficult temperament, parenting stress, and early-mother-infant interaction. *Norwegian Journal of Psychiatry, 60*, 379–386.

McFarland, J., Salisbury, A., Battle, C., Hawes, K., Halloran, K., & Lester, B. (2011). Major depressive disorder during pregnancy and emotional attachment to the fetus. *Archives of Women's Mental Health, 14*, 425–434.

Muzik, M., Bocknek, E. L., Broderick, A., Richardson, P., Rosenblum, K. L., Thelen, K., & Seng, J. S. (2013). Mother-infant bonding impairment across the first 6 months postpartum: The primacy of psychopathology in women with childhood abuse and neglect histories. *Archives of Women's Mental Health, 16*(1), 29–38. doi:10.1007/s00737-012-0312-0

O'Hara, M., & McCabe, J. (2013). Postpartum depression: Current status and future directions. *Annual Review of Clinical Psychology, 9*, 379–407.

Olson, A. L., Dietric, A. J., Prazar, G., & Hurley, J. (2006). Brief maternal depression screening at well-child visits. *Pediatrics, 118*(1), 207–216.

Radesky, J., Zukerman, B., Silverstein, M., Rivara, F., Barr, M., Taylor, J., . . . Barr, R. (2013). Inconsolable infant crying and maternal postpartum depressive symptoms. *Pediatrics, 131*, e1857.

Radye-Yarrow, M., Martinez, P., Mayfield, A., & Ronsaville, D. (1998). *Children of Depressed Mothers: From Early Childhood to Maturity*. New York: Cambridge University Press.

Rafferty, Y., Griffin, K., & Robokos, D. (2010). Maternal depression and parental distress among families in the early head start research and evaluation project: Risk factors within the family setting. *Infant Mental Health Journal, 31*(5), 543–569.

Rifkin-Graboi, A., Borelli, J., & Enlow, M. (2009). Neurobiology of stress in infancy. In C. Zeanah (Ed.), Handbook of Infant Mental Health (3rd ed., Ch. 4, pp. 59–81). New York: The Guilford Press.

Rosenblum, K., Dayton, C., & Muzik, M. (2009). Infant social and emotional development. In C. Zeanah (Ed.), *Handbook of Infant Mental Health* (3rd ed.). New York, NY: The Guilford Press.

Rothbart, M. (2011). *Becoming Who We Are: Temperment and Personality in Development*. New York: The Guilford Press.

Simpson, T. Condon, E., Price, R., Finch, B., Sadler, L., & Ordway, M. (2015). Demystifying infant mental health: What the primary provider needs to know. *Journal of Pediatric Health Care, 30*(1), 38–48.

Slade, A., Cohen, L., Sadler, L., & Miller, M. (2009). The psychology and psychopathology of pregnancy. In C. Zeanah (Ed.), *Handbook of Infant Mental Health* (3rd ed., Ch. 5, pp. 80–103). New York: The Guilford Press.

Stowe, Z. (2012). *Psychopharmacology during Pregnancy and Lactation*. Paper presented at the Oakstone Institute Psychiatry Board Review Course, March 15, 2012. Purchased as a set from www.CMEinfo.com; Oakstone Publishing, LLC.

Wan, M., & Green, J. (2009). The impact of maternal psychopathology on child-mother attachment. *Archives of Women's Mental Health, 12*, 123–134.

Yurdakul, Z., Akman, I., Kuscu, K., Karabekiroglu, A., Yalah, G., Demir, F., & Ozek, E. (2009). Maternal psychological problems associated with neonatal intensive care admission. *International Journal of Pediatrics*. Retrieved from https://www.hindawi.com/journals/ijpedi/2009/591359/

Zeanah, C., & Zeanah, P. (2009). The scope of infant mental health. In C. Zeanah (Ed.), *Handbook of Infant Mental Health* (3rd ed., Ch. 1, pp. 5–21). New York: The Guilford Press.

Chapter 4

New Fatherhood

An Overview of Men's Perinatal Mental Health

Daniel B. Singley and Lisa M. Edwards

New Fatherhood: An Overview of Men's Perinatal Mental Health

Similar to stereotypes regarding the role of mothers, there are also stereotypes and role expectations concerning the transition to fatherhood. Although it is a cultural norm for fathers to be involved in the birth and care of their infants, there is still a pervasive belief that parenting an infant is restricted to "mothering." This perspective greatly short-changes the role of fathers. There are clear benefits that children, mothers and fathers experience when new fathers are intricately involved with their families and become fully engaged in the care of their children and newborns. Men commonly experience a very rich psychological transition as they become fathers, but like mothers, they can experience perinatal stress and mental health concerns.

Emerging literature recognizes that the transition to parenthood has an impact on men and that men can be at risk of developing postpartum depression. Unfortunately, given the lack of awareness about paternal postpartum depression, fathers are infrequently screened and diagnosed, and rarely treated (Musser, Ahmed, Foli, & Coddington, 2013). Paternal postpartum depression has consequences for the father, father–infant bond, infant mental health, as well as a host of other negative long-term psychosocial outcomes in children (Berger, Carlson, Bzostek, & Osborne, 2008; Bronte-Tinkew, Moore, Matthews, & Carrano, 2007). In this chapter, the authors will review the literature on the psychological transition to fatherhood and discuss key considerations and suggestions regarding how health care providers can most effectively engage new fathers in treatment.

Shift in Father's Role

The 1990s were dubbed "the decade of the disappearing father," due to the high number of U.S. children living apart from their biological fathers (Blankenhorn, 1995). In contrast, the current decade could be dubbed "the decade of the reappearing father" because there has been emerging recognition, research, policy and resources dedicated to promoting the importance of fathers in the well-being of their children and partners (M. E. Lamb, 2010). This shift in recognizing fatherhood was reflected in President Obama's statement in his *Responsible Fatherhood and Strong Communities Initiative.* In his initiative, President Obama recognized the important role of fathers: "We need fathers to realize that responsibility does not end at conception. We need [fathers] to realize that what makes you a man is not the ability to have a child—it is the courage to raise one."

Unfortunately, many men lack clear guidance and role models that teach them how to be engaged, active fathers. This lack of guidance leads to cognitive, behavioral and psychological issues that often go unrecognized until a crisis emerges. Compounding this issue is men's difficulty in connecting with their internal experience when problems arise (Berger et al., 2008), and men's historical underutilization of mental health services (Vogel, Wester, Hammer, & Downing-Matibag, 2014).

Michael Lamb (1995), an expert in the psychology of fatherhood, argued that there is a shift in the popular understanding of the fatherhood role (Lamb, 1995). According to Lamb, the phases of fatherhood in the United States have gone from the "moral father" modeling Christian values and living during Puritan times (Demos, 1982), to a focus on breadwinner during the industrialization of the mid-nineteenth century (Pleck, 1976). The dawn of the Second World War brought a focus on fathers as serving as a gender role model, in particular for boys. In the late 1960s, for the first time, social norms began to shift toward identifying that fathers need to be active and nurturing caretakers of their children. The fundamentals of "good fathering" identified in the late 1960s persist today. These fundamentals include moral development, providing resources, and serving as a gender role—and more recently include direct caretaking of their very young babies.

The Transition to Fatherhood

The physical and emotional adjustment to fatherhood can be complex and demanding (Kim & Swain, 2007; Lara, Navarro, & Navarrete, 2010; Sheng, Le, & Perry, 2010). Caring for an infant's needs can be exhausting, and new parents commonly experience continual sleep deprivation. Furthermore, the added stress of time away from work can increase anxiety. The father's relationship with his partner commonly changes in dramatic ways, requiring that the mother and father deal with new "family operational" aspects of caring for themselves and their new baby along with the psychosocial changes of new parenthood.

Many new fathers wrestle with gender role conflict, or men's experience of "rigid, sexist, or restrictive gender roles, learned during socialization, [which] result in the personal restriction, devaluation, or violation of others or self" (O'Neil, 1990, p. 25). Fathers experiencing this type of conflict commonly have difficulty engaging in behaviors such as cooing, soothing, hugging, and playing with their infants—and sons in particular—due to deep-seated beliefs that these behaviors are feminine or "weak." In this way, fathers who experience high levels of gender role conflict have concerns that they will be perceived as feminine. Men also are commonly socialized to express "acceptable" masculine emotions such as anger. When new fathers experience stress during the transition to fatherhood, they may be more likely to channel their frustration by withdrawing from the child and/or partner, which can ultimately result in a decreased father–child attachment bond (Levant, 1995).

David and Brannon (1976) distilled the essence of masculine socialization from a variety of research and theory by positing that the four broad themes of traditional masculinity in the United States are:

- Anti-femininity—"No sissy stuff."
- Status and Achievement—"Be the big wheel."
- Inexpressiveness and Independence—"The sturdy oak."
- Adventurousness and Aggressiveness—"Give 'em hell."

Absent from these themes are some essential elements for the effective parenting of babies and children, including nurturance, warmth, emotional awareness, and working as a team with mothers. Fathers who feel bound to male gender role stereotypes may be reluctant to strap on a Baby Björn, pack up the diaper bag, and head to a play group with other dads. Furthermore, both men and women receive this socialization about what it means to be a man and, more specifically, the father of an infant (Parke, 1996). In this way, both the father and his wife might simultaneously feel the need to have the father more involved with his infant, while unknowingly putting up barriers for him to do so due to outdated beliefs about "what makes a man." Furthermore, fathers who experience difficulty juggling work-life balance demands in the perinatal period may opt to enact the provider role and experience a sense of competence by increasing their time spent at work. This imbalance results in decreased involvement with their babies, along with a concomitant increase in their partner's management of childcare responsibilities and a reduction in the father's sense of competence in caring for his child.

New fathers' attentiveness to their children also may be related to changes in hormonal levels that mirror those of mothers throughout the perinatal period, specifically, increased levels of prolactin, cortisol and estrogen (estradiol) with decreased levels of testosterone around the birth of their infants (Storey, Walsh, Quinton, & Wynne-Edwards, 2000). Each of these hormones has implications for different aspects of how men behave with their newborns and partners, suggesting that imbalances in these levels may account for psychological and/or behavioral issues. Although there is as of yet no research definitively linking these phenomena, there is some initial evidence that perinatal depression may have a biological basis, potentially linked to changes in hormone levels (Ramchandani, Stein, Evans, & O'Connor, 2005).

The "Fatherhood Generation Gap"

Gender roles in the United States are trending toward equality, and perspectives on fatherhood have therefore likewise evolved. Currently, fathers are expected to engage in higher levels of involvement in domestic duties, including caring for babies. Additionally, it is important to understand that the current generation of young fathers (i.e., Generations "X and Y" born in the 1970s–1990s) may experience a kind of fatherhood socialization *generation gap*. On the one hand, these men have seen the evolution of the father's role in sharing more responsibility for caretaking and financial responsibilities. On the other hand, they have also been influenced by their baby boomer generation fathers' tendency to serve as gender role models rather than as direct caretakers (Duncombe & Marsden, 1999; Hochschild, 1994). These fathers may experience pressure to adhere to persistent, traditional male gender norms such as the "sturdy oak" and "big wheel" (David & Brannon, 1976), which influence most men in current society. Furthermore, contemporary new fathers are much more likely to have partners who work outside the home as compared to fathers in the latter half of the 20th century (Occupational Outlook Handbook, 2015). As Silverstein, Auerbach, and Levant (2002) noted, fathers who have been socialized to focus narrowly on their role in providing resources to their families, but who are not the sole provider of those resources for their families are "feeling all of the disadvantages of the role and none of the satisfaction." (Silverstein et al., 2002, p. 362). The information in this section underscores research and theory which shows that the new generation of fathers is expected to be highly involved in the caregiving of their infants. At the same time, they are caught in a type of "fatherhood generation gap," which may result in challenges and potentially mental health difficulties as they work to manage their new role as fathers.

Research on Fatherhood Involvement

Paternal involvement was first defined by Lamb, Pleck, Charnov, and Levine (1987) and the most common model of involvement consists of three factors: engagement, availability and accessibility, and responsibility (McKelley & Rochlen, 2015). Engagement refers to activities such as playing games, reading/telling stories, telling the child they are loved, and so on (Waller, 2012). Availability reflects the extent to which the father is accessible to the child and is often measured regarding the time spent with the child. Responsibility indicates the degree to which the father is involved in the day-to-day decisions such as medical checkups and attending parent–teacher conferences. Fathers' involvement with their infants has been shown to have a host of positive outcomes for children, mothers, and fathers alike (Parke, 1996; J. H. Pleck, 2010). Children whose fathers are highly involved with them, especially from birth, have been shown to be more emotionally secure and confident in exploring their environment. This emotional connection with their father leads to having better social relationships with peers as they grow older (Yeung, Duncan, & Hill, 2000). These children are also less likely to get in trouble at home, school or in the neighborhood (Harris, Furstenberg, & Marmer, 1998). Fathers spend a considerably higher percentage of their time alone with their infants in highly stimulating, playful interactions (Parke, 1996), and, by playing with dad, their children learn how to regulate their feelings and behavior (Fletcher, 2011). For example, rough-and-tumble play with dad can a be a way in which children learn about appropriately managing aggressive interactions and physical contact without losing control of their emotions. Figure 4.1 emphasizes another means through which fathers' involvement with their babies may relate to the child's subsequent mental health functioning.

Essentially, fathers stereotypically have highly arousing yet shorter "bursts" of interaction with their babies (think of a father tossing his baby in the air several times and then setting her or him down), while mothers commonly have more sustained lower-intensity interactions with them (feeding, reading, rocking, soothing). The benefit from the father's play style is that it gives the baby repeated opportunities to calm down to baseline from a highly aroused state on their own. Over time, this experience may impact the development of the child's ability to self-soothe and regulate emotion.

Many new fathers may question their competence as a parent, and they may lack parenting self-efficacy beliefs (Coleman & Karraker, 1997). Social Cognitive Theory posits that self-efficacy for a certain behavior—for example, caring for an infant—is one of the strongest determinants of whether or

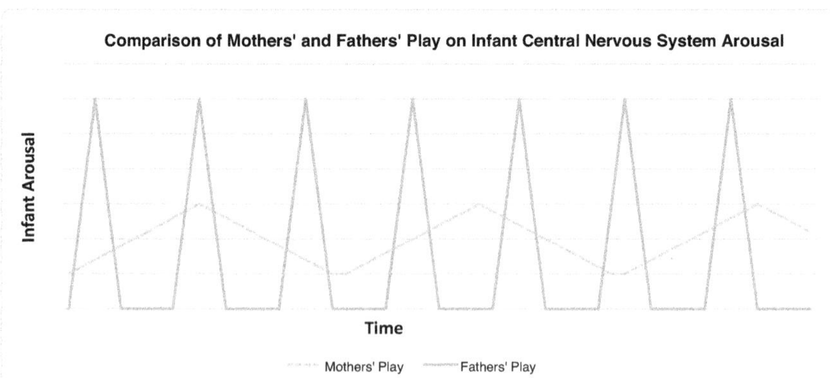

Figure 4.1 Comparison of Mothers' and Fathers' Play on Infant Central Nervous System Arousal

not a person will attempt a given behavior (Bandura, 1986). A variety of research has shown that the more stress and marital dissatisfaction a new father experiences, the lower his paternal self-efficacy and, therefore, his direct involvement with his infant (Murdock, 2013; Sevigny & Loutzenhiser, 2010). Furthermore, spousal/partner support in the form of "other-efficacy" describes that how a man's wife perceives his ability to parent an infant also likely informs a new father's self-efficacy. Spousal support predicts higher levels of psychological well-being, parental effectiveness and coping (Aycan & Eskin, 2005). While many mothers encourage fathers to be involved, one study found that the majority of women did not want their partners to be more involved with their children, even while 40% of fathers wanted to spend more time with their children than they currently were spending (Quinn & Staines, 1979). This tendency in mothers is referred to as a "gatekeeping" role, and research has shown that mothers' views of their role as caregiver and that of the father draw heavily to bear on the father's level of involvement with his children (McBride et al., 2005). In this way, many factors may influence a father's self-efficacy, or lack thereof, during the transition to fatherhood—and that both his own and his partner's sense of confidence in his ability to parent play a strong role in how, when, and if he is involved with his baby.

While the majority of research in the psychology of early childhood has focused on attachment theory (e.g., Bowlby, Ainsworth, Main), researchers in this area rarely factor in the father as an important attachment figure. Although John Bowlby himself posited that children need at least one positive attachment figure, neither he nor any of the investigators currently doing work in this area have shown that mothers are superior to fathers regarding caring for young babies or fostering securely attached children. Because there are some documented ways in which fathers tend to interact differently with their children (such as the "jazzed up" playing style described above), several researchers over the past 20 years have begun to tease out father-specific ways that men make unique contributions to their children's development. The paternal activation relationship line of research (Demontigny, Girard, Lacharite, Dubeau, & Devault, 2013; Grossmann et al., 2002; Paquette, 2004) capitalizes on the tendency for fathers to serve as guides to the outside world (Rosenberg & Wilcox, 2006) and to engage in controlled risk-taking along with their children. As opposed to the Strange Situation assessment (examining attachment), researchers assess the paternal activation relationship using a "risky situation" methodology in which the father goes along with his toddler. In this approach, researchers identify the extent to which the child (in the presence of her or his father) can engage in a series of controlled "risky" situations along with the father. In this way, the need to return to a safe attachment figure is obviated by the child's sense of comfort in continuing to explore novel and/or concerning situations *along with her or his father.*

Another element of parenthood has focused on the mother's experience of the timing of pregnancy and becoming a parent. Women 35 years old and older are often considered to have a "biological clock" that ostensibly increases their desire to have children as they age. Wendy Goldberg (2014) conducted a study addressing the concept that fathers experience a social "clock" that predisposes them to enter into fatherhood at different periods of their lives as well (Goldberg, 2014). Among her findings from this "social clock" perspective, so-called on-time fathers who followed traditional age norms for becoming a father adapted most readily to parenthood. Younger fathers tended to evidence higher levels of neuroticism, which reflects negative emotions and emotional instability. On the other hand, older, delayed-timing fathers were shown to have personality characteristics such as openness to new experiences, which predict higher-quality parenting (Cooney, Pedersen, Indelicato, & Palkovitz, 1993). This line of research suggests the need to address the father's characteristics to understand his transition to parenthood.

The information in this section illustrates how a man's fatherhood role is but one of many elements of his masculine socialization, and that the shaping of that role is ongoing throughout his life. It is essential for practitioners to recognize that men experiencing a disconnect between a more traditional male gender role and the contemporary expectations of generative fathering behavior during the perinatal period may experience distress. This distress may result in a father's withdrawal from his partner and infant, and in some cases, may lead to the development of mental health concerns such as anxiety and depression. The complex interaction of fatherhood/gender role conflict, partner social support, paternal involvement, self-efficacy, and mental health problems represent a fertile area for practitioners to assist men navigating the transition to fatherhood. Importantly, it also calls attention to ways in which professionals working with men might prevent and treat mental health concerns.

Men's Perinatal Mental Health

As with other periods of developmental change for men (e.g., puberty, marriage, divorce, death of a loved one, retirement), the transition to fatherhood brings with it an attendant level of stress. Due to the stressful nature of the transition to fatherhood, men may also experience a heightened risk perinatal mood and anxiety disorders (PMAD) similar to the maternal PMADs described in Chapter 2. As noted above, the majority of research and theory about perinatal mental health focuses on mothers and, to a lesser extent, children—while addressing the entire newly expanded family system, it is essential to consider the father's mental health as well. It is important first to address how masculine identity development—the foundation upon which the father and partner roles are built—affects men throughout the perinatal period.

Alexithymia and Masked Male Depression

Except mood- and relationship-focused mental health issues that present during the perinatal period, few if any father-specific forms of mental health issues have received much attention in research. However, alexithymia and masked male depression reflect two key concepts for mental health practitioners to understand to work with and conceptualize men making the transition to fatherhood.

Alexithymia reflects "a specific disturbance in psychic functioning characterized by difficulties in the capacity to verbalize affect and to elaborate fantasies" (Taylor, 1984, p. 725). Alexithymia describes the phenomenon in which some men and women (although it is observed more commonly in males) have considerable difficulty in connecting to and discussing their emotional experiences. Men who have psychological disorders and who experience alexithymia often also have a comorbid psychosomatic illness, psychogenic pain, substance abuse, anxiety, and depression—albeit with an extremely limited ability to verbalize these experiences. Given the overwhelming focus on a mother's mental health during the perinatal period along with the common advice to "just support your partner," alexithymia reflects another component that serves to keep new and expectant fathers' mental health issues off the radars of practitioners, partners, friends and even themselves.

Rabinowitz and Cochran (2008) initially posited the existence of Male Masked Depression (MMD) as a means to deepen clinicians' understanding of a type of mood disorders that may be harder to detect than typical Unipolar Depressive Disorder (Rabinowitz & Cochran, 2008). These authors posit that MMD reflects a longer-term, and the more insidious onset of depression that may be overlooked as health care providers focus on more immediate presenting concerns such as relationship issues, transitional stress, and substance abuse to name a few. In essence, rather than appearing weepy or overly depressed, men suffering from MMD commonly evidence a tendency to self-isolate, use substances and express anger or irritability. If compounded with alexithymia and the general male tendency to avoid mental health help-seeking, male patients experiencing this type of mood issue may languish in an ongoing way due a lack of recognition of their own MMD symptoms.

Postpartum Depression (PPD)

Paternal postpartum depression has been defined in various ways in research and clinical practice, as there are no existing diagnostic criteria for this mental health concern (Kim & Swain, 2007). As discussed in Chapter 2, with the creation of DSM-5 postpartum depression was changed to include a "with peripartum onset" modifier to include the timeframe during pregnancy (APA, 2013). Although the DSM definition of depressive disorders with peripartum is restricted to 4 weeks postpartum, most often perinatal depression is expanded to include up to 1 year postpartum. It should be noted that although depression may look different among men because it is "masked" (hidden) through expressions of irritability, anger or withdrawal (Cochran & Rabinowitz, 2000), the DSM-5 does not have any specifiers to recognize and account for the masculine-specific expressions of depression.

For most research about maternal and paternal PPD, the Edinburgh Postnatal Depression Scale (Heim et al., 2000; EPDS) is the most widely used scale. This measure consists of 10 self-report items about depressive and anxiety symptoms. Cut-off scores are employed to note depression, and support for its psychometric properties with both women and men exist (Kim & Swain, 2007; Matthey, Barnett, Kavanagh, & Howie, 2001). Other self-report measures for PPD have included the Beck Depression Inventory-II (BDI-II; (Beck, Steer, & Brown, 1996), and the CES-D (Radloff, 1977), though the EPDS remains the most common.

As a result of differing methods of diagnosis (Gawlik et al., 2014), differing timing of measurements, and small samples (Paulson & Bazemore, 2010; Roubinov, Luecken, Crnic & Gonzales, 2014), estimates of paternal postpartum depression have varied from 1% to 26% within the United States (Goodman, 2004; Ramchandani et al., 2005). In the only meta-analysis that is published about paternal perinatal depression, Paulson and Bazemore (2010) reviewed 43 studies from 16 countries to estimate paternal depression rates between the first trimester and 1 year postpartum (Paulson & Bazemore, 2010). These authors found an overall rate of paternal depression during this period to be 10.4%. In comparison to the 4.8% 12-month prevalence base rate of depression for men in the United States (Kessler et al., 2003), the findings of the meta-analysis provide additional support for the importance of attending to men's perinatal mental health needs.

The Paulson and Bazemore (2010) meta-analysis revealed additional findings of interest (Paulson & Bazemore, 2010). First, the incidence of postpartum depression for men was greatest between the initial 3 and 6 months of fatherhood, although the authors note that the small number of studies included in this analysis suggest the findings should be interpreted with caution. Previous studies have found that fathers tend to suffer from depressive symptoms more frequently prenatally compared to postpartum (Boyce, Condon, Barton, & Corkindale, 2007; Buist, Morse, & Durkin, 2003; Condon, Boyce, & Corkindale, 2004), implying the prenatal period was most stressful for men. Further research is needed to understand better the nature of prenatal depression and its course throughout the postpartum period among fathers.

Prevalence of Other PMADs

Rates for other perinatal mood and anxiety disorders among fathers are difficult to obtain, though there have been a few studies to explore these. For example, a range of 0% to 4.7% has been found for paternal postpartum

PTSD (Ayers, Wright, & Wells, 2007; Bradley, Slade, & Leviston, 2008). For paternal postpartum anxiety, rates have varied from 4.4% to 9.7% (Bradley et al., 2008; S. Matthey, Barnett, Howie, & Kavanagh, 2003). In a recent study of Obsessive-Compulsive Disorder in fathers, authors found a prevalence of 3.4% in the third trimester and 1.8% in the postpartum period (Coelho et al., 2014). Finally, a study of depression and bipolar disorder (Pinheiro et al., 2011) suggests that depressive episodes were significantly associated with manic/hypomanic episodes for fathers during pregnancy and up to 12 months post-delivery. For example, among the 5% of fathers who were diagnosed as depressed during the prenatal period, 2.1% of them also experienced manic episodes and 3.3% experienced hypomanic episodes. Clearly much more research is needed to understand better the prevalence and comorbidity of these mental health disorders and how they change over time during the perinatal period.

Risk Factors for Postpartum Depression

The Parental Alliance

It is a well-established finding that a couple's relationship satisfaction decreases significantly after the birth of their first child, in large part due to role conflicts and restrictions in their freedom (Twenge, Campbell, & Foster, 2003). The fact that mothers' experiences of perinatal mental health issues such as depression is a strong predictor of men's mental health problems (Condon et al., 2004) is a testament to how key the parental alliance is for the health of the family system. In a recent study addressing how this relationship may be linked, researchers found that maternal and paternal postpartum depression were indirectly related through pathways of impaired spousal support and reduced relationship satisfaction (Don, & Mickelson, 2012). It seems clear that new fathers need to give *and* receive support from their partners to thrive during the transition to parenthood. It is also a clear indicator that clinicians should evaluate both mothers and fathers for mental health issues whenever possible.

Poor relationship satisfaction has been found to be a risk factor in other recent studies about paternal depression (Gawlik et al., 2014; Wee, Skouteris, Pier, Richardson & Milgrom, 2011). Importantly, in the Gawlik et al. study, birth concerns and relationship quality were found to be more important in predicting postpartum depression among fathers than were prenatal depressive symptoms. Depressive disorders among fathers are associated with increased risk of inter-parental conflict (P. G. Ramchandani et al., 2011), and decreased relationship quality and decreased co-parenting (Bronte-Tinkew et al., 2007). Again, some of these latter findings suggest associations between these variables and do not indicate causation.

Lack of Social Support

The perinatal period reflects a period of heightened stress during which men may benefit from increased social support; however, men are typically socialized to rely heavily on their intimate partner for the majority of their emotional support (Fischer & Good, 1997). Fathers who maintain solid social support networks experience a buffer from the conflicts and demands associated with parenting, while also providing role models which facilitate a sense of competence as parents (Aycan & Eskin, 2005). However, as both parents increase their focus on the needs of their new child, men are often less proactive about seeking out social support from sources other than their partner due to increased demands of managing a new baby (Patulny, 2011). This decrease in outside support sets the stage for added stress and isolation, which may ultimately place undue strain on the relationship with his spouse, further isolation from mother and child, and limited ability to experience good caretaking experiences with his child and increased self-efficacy beliefs (Paquette, 2004).

While the parental alliance is one highly important element in a man's transition to fatherhood, it is critically important that both parents continue to nurture their broader networks of support to buffer and reduce the impact of the stress of birth and new parenting (Crnic, Friedrich, & Greenberg, 1983). In the rush of friends and family to meet the new baby, men are likely to remain largely focused on the mother and baby, even to the exclusion of involvement in activities with others of which they typically find energizing (e.g., "She's up all night with the baby—I can't ask to play golf."). Women are commonly the "Social Chairs" in a partnership, and men tend not to reach out to others as often, particularly if one is a father but the other is childless.

Outcomes of Postpartum Depression

The effects of perinatal depression can be seen in fathers, their children, and the parenting relationship (J. Paulson, Dauber, & Leiferman, 2006). In a large study of depressed fathers and their infants (Bronte-Tinkew et al., 2007), fathers who were depressed had less frequent engagement with their children and were less likely to engage in enrichment activities (e.g., singing, reading and telling stories) with their children. In a study that further explored mediators through which father's postnatal depression was associated with emotional-behavioral difficulties in their children, irritable parenting behaviors (e.g., yelling and losing one's temper) emerged as a significant variable (Giallo, Cooklin, Wade, D'Esposito, & Nicholson, 2014).

Researchers have found that children whose fathers have postpartum depression tend to demonstrate increased behavioral problems, including hyperactivity and conduct problems (Ramchandani et al., 2005). The children of fathers who reported depressive symptoms when they were infants had poorer outcomes (e.g., increased hyperactivity, peer problems and conduct concerns) at age 4–5 years (Bronte-Tinkew et al., 2007).

Treating Paternal Postpartum Depression

Regardless of setting, all providers should work to engage fathers fully in perinatal services, including screening for mental health concerns. At the broadest level, practitioners need to recognize that men in the perinatal period are at an elevated risk for mental health issues (Ramchandani et al., 2005), yet the majority of scholarly and clinical work in this area focuses on mothers' and the infants' well-being (Brockington, 2004). A key challenge for clinicians is to be aware of the unconscious gendered stereotypes (e.g., "dads' primary role is to support mom") that they may perpetuate as a result of socialization regarding gender and parental roles. Concrete training in the psychology of men and masculinity is not commonly incorporated into graduate training or continuing education programming in psychology, so many practitioners are ill-prepared to recognize or to support men regarding common issues such as perinatal depression as they make the transition to fatherhood. For example, masked male depression commonly manifests as anger/irritation, substance use, and withdrawal, so psychologists need to familiarize themselves with the presentation and dynamics that support this maladaptive tendency to "stuff" difficult experiences (Rabinowitz & Cochran, 2008). Men are socialized not to ask for help, and while it is particularly difficult to do so during a period in which they believe they need to support and provide for their partner, it can be very helpful to emphasize the need to take care of themselves to present the best version of themselves. Developing a greater awareness of masculine socialization, the psychology of early fatherhood, and men's perinatal mental health issues will enable clinicians to work more efficiently with this at-risk population.

Another recommendation would be to include regular screenings for new and expectant fathers—in particular when either the father or mother has a history of any mental health concern (Hynan, Mounts, & Vanderbilt, 2013). As noted earlier, nearly 10% of men experience perinatal depression (Paulson & Bazemore, 2010), but they are not screened for mental health issues during antenatal or well-baby visits postpartum (Spector, 2006). Using a validated screening tool such as the Edinburg Postnatal Depression Scale (Cox, Holden, & Sagovsky, 1987) to assess the fathers during this period would increase early identification of fathers having difficulty (Hynan et al., 2013). In practice, this would mean screening patients who are new or expectant fathers, as well as working to schedule conjoint office visits to assess the male partners of new mothers (e.g., the "primary patient"). The American Academy of Pediatrics (Earls, et al., 2010) recommends that pediatricians assess mothers for postpartum depression at 1-, 2-, 4-, and 6- month follow-up visits. The National Perinatal Association (Hynan et al., 2013) recommends that fathers be screened at least twice for postpartum depression during the first postpartum year. As a result of fathers' perinatal depression being more likely to develop around 3–6 months postpartum (Paulson & Bazemore, 2010), clinicians should also keep an eye toward assessing new fathers' mental health issues during this period.

It is also important to educate new parents about the reality that parents commonly experience regarding decreased relationship satisfaction immediately after the birth of a child (Twenge et al., 2003). New fathers can benefit from concrete guidance regarding the need to actively engage their partners on an emotional level about any issues they are experiencing. By avoiding the tendency to ignore or "power through" difficulties they may be having, men can work proactively to schedule regular weekly "check-ins" to discuss how they are doing with their partners. Teaching new parents to use basic assertive communication skills such as leading with open questions, making restatements, and avoiding the "fix-it" approach is an excellent way to foster higher levels of relationship satisfaction and shared understanding.

Finally, fathers tend to have lower parenting self-efficacy than mothers (Hudson, Elek, & Fleck, 2001), and lower self-efficacy has been shown to relate to parenting stress, depressive symptoms, and partner relational functioning (Sevigny & Loutzenhiser, 2010). Therefore, it is important for fathers to enhance their parenting self-efficacy. One way this can be accomplished is by encouraging fathers to engage in as much of the direct caretaking of their infant (e.g., soothing, swaddling, bathing, burping) as soon as possible. Having a frank discussion with new mothers and fathers regarding their perceptions about specific areas of concern regarding his ability to care for their baby is an excellent way to discern areas of higher and lower parenting self-efficacy. Another way that fathers can connect with their partners and build confidence even before the baby is born is to obtain a birth plan template (for an example from the American Pregnancy Association, see: http://americanpregnancy.org/labor-and-birth/birth-plan/) and interview mom to clarify a "decision tree" for the day of the birth. Dads can also take the lead on gathering information about pediatricians, interviewing their partner about preferences, and doing an initial round of calls to see about interviewing pediatricians.

Summary

Practitioners in a variety of settings including OB clinics, birth centers, pediatrics, perinatology, social work, psychiatry and psychology are more likely than ever to be in contact with new and expectant fathers throughout the perinatal period. Practitioners who work with fathers in the perinatal period can assist in their transition to fatherhood by creating programs that are targeted toward their unique needs. While the research on fatherhood engagement programs has matured considerably in the past 20 years (for two excellent reviews of this literature, see Rosenberg & Wilcox, 2006; Panter-Brick et al., 2014), there has been relatively little focus on programmatic efforts aimed at new or expectant fathers. One notable exception is the *Boot Camp for New Dads* program, which is conducted in a variety of cities throughout the country. Results from a 2012 study of postpartum fathers who completed this class during the pregnancy period experienced significant gains in confidence regarding becoming a father, creating a parenting team with the baby's mother, and bonding with the baby (Miller, 2012).

> When developing and implementing a fatherhood engagement and education program, it is essential to understand the unique needs of the population in question. Bronte-Tinkew et al. (2007) studied effective elements of evidence-based interventions for fathers and concluded that some of the key factors of "what works" in such programs include:
>
> - Incorporating teaching methods and materials that are appropriate for fathers and the cultures of the populations
> - Selecting and recruiting staff who are experienced, empathetic and well-connected in the community
> - Using curricula targeted around a few core issues, and which have been shown to be effective in influencing parenting behaviors
> - Using a variety of teaching methods to focus on fathers and personalize the information

The parenting program that has to date received the most rigorous evaluation regarding randomized control trials is the "Triple P" Positive Parenting Program developed by Matthew Sanders (Sanders, 1999). While not specifically focused on fathers, this program blends seminars, group sessions and individual sessions which have been shown to result in a variety of positive outcomes for children, parents and families as-a-whole. The flexible format of the Triple P program allows a single practitioner to provide this program to interested parents, or on a larger scale institutions and organizations may implement this approach.

References

American Psychiatric Association, A. P. (Ed.) (2000). *Diagnostic Criteria From DSM-IV-TR* (4th ed.). Arlington, VA: Author.

American Psychiatric Association. (Ed.) (2013). *DSM-5 Criteria.* Arlington, VA: Author.

Aycan, Z., & Eskin, M. (2005). Childcare, spousal, and organizational support in predicting work-family conflict for females and males in dual-earner families with preschool children. *Sex Roles, 53*, 453–471.

Ayers, S., Wright, D. B., & Wells, N. (2007). Symptoms of post-traumatic stress disorder in couples after birth: Association with the couple's relationship and parent-baby bond. *Journal of Reproductive and Infant Psychology, 25*, 40–50.

Bandura, A. (1986). *Social Foundations of Thought and Action: A Social Cognitive Theory*. Englewood Cliffs, NJ: Prentice-Hall.
Beck, A. T., Steer, R. A., & Brown, G. K. (1996). *Manual for Beck Depression Inventory-II*. San Antonio, TX: Psychological Corporation.
Berger, L. M., Carlson, M. J., Bzostek, S. H., & Osborne, C. (2008). Parenting practices of resident fathers: The role of marital and biological ties. *Journal of Marriage and Family, 70*, 625–639.
Blankenhorn, D. (1995). *Fatherless America: Confronting Our Most Urgent Social Problem*. New York, NY: Basic Books.
Boyce, P., Condon, J., Barton, J., & Corkindale, C. (2007). First-time fathers study: Psychological distress in expectant fathers during pregnancy. *Australian & New Zealand Journal of Psychiatry, 41*, 718–725.
Bradley, R., Slade, P., & Leviston, A. (2008). Low rates of PTSD in men attending childbirth: A preliminary study. *British Journal of Clinical Psychology, 47*, 295–302.
Brockington, I. (2004). Postpartum psychiatric disorders. *The Lancet, 363*, 303–310.
Bronte-Tinkew, J., Moore, K. A., Matthews, G., & Carrano, J. (2007). Symptoms of major depression in a sample of fathers of infants sociodemographic correlates and links to father involvement. *Journal of Family Issues, 28*, 61–99.
Buist, A., Morse, C. A., & Durkin, S. (2003). Men's adjustment to fatherhood: Implications for obstetric health care. *Journal of Obstetric, Gynecologic, & Neonatal Nursing, 32*, 172–180.
Cochran, S. V., & Rabinowitz, F. E. (2000). *Men and Depression: Clinical and Empirical Perspectives*. San Diego, CA: Academic Press.
Coelho, F. M., da Silva, R. A. A., Quevedo, L., Souza, L. D., Pinheiro, K. A., & Pinheiro, R. T. (2014). Obsessive-compulsive disorder in fathers during pregnancy and postpartum. *Revista Brasileira de Psiquiatria, 36*, 272–272.
Coleman, P. K., & Karraker, K. H. (1997). Self-efficacy and parenting quality: Findings and future applications. *Developmental Review, 18*, 47–85.
Condon, T. J., Boyce, P., & Corkindale, C. J. (2004). The first-time fathers study: A prospective study of the mental health and wellbeing of men during the transition to parenthood. *Australian and New Zealand Journal of Psychiatry, 38*, 56–64.
Cooney, T. M., Pedersen, F. A., Indelicato, S., & Palkovitz, R. (1993). Timing of fatherhood: Is "on-time" optimal? *Journal of Marriage and the Family, 55*, 205–215.
Cox, J. L., Holden, J. M., & Sagovsky, R. (1987). Detection of postnatal depression: Development of the 10-item Edinburgh Postnatal Depression Scale. *The British Journal of Psychiatry, 150*, 782–786.
Crnic, K. A., Friedrich, W. N., & Greenberg, M. T. (1983). Adaptation of families with mentally retarded children: A model of stress, coping, and family ecology. *American Journal of Mental Deficiency, 88*, 125–138.
David, S. D., & Brannon, R. (1976). *The Forty-Nine Percent Majority: The Male Sex Role*. Reading, MA: Addison Wesley Publishing Company.
Demontigny, F., Girard, M. E., Lacharite, C., Dubeau, D., & Devault, A. (2013). Psychosocial factors associated with paternal postnatal depression. *Journal of Affective Disorders, 150*(1), 44–49. doi:10.1016/j.jad.2013.01.048
Demos, J. (1982). The changing faces of fatherhood: A new exploration in American family history. In S. H. Cath, A. R. Gurwitt, & J. M. Ross (Eds.), *Father and Child: Developmental and Clinical Perspectives* (pp. 425–445). Boston: Little, Brown.

Don, P. B., & Mickelson, K. D. (2012). Paternal postpartum depression: The role of maternal postpartum depression, spousal support, and relationship satisfaction. *Couple and Family Psychology: Research and Practice, 1*(4), 323–334.

Duncombe, J., & Marsden, D. (1999). Love and intimacy: The gender division of emotion and "emotion work": A neglected aspect of sociological discussion of heterosexual relationships. In G. Allan (Ed.), *The Sociology of the Family: A Reader* (pp. 91–110). Malden, MA: Blackwell.

Earls, M. F., Committee on Psychosocial Aspects of Child & Family Health American Academy of Pediatrics. (2010). Incorporating recognition and management of perinatal and postpartum depression into pediatric practice. *Pediatrics, 126*(5), 1032–1039. doi:10.1542/peds.2010-2348

Fischer, A. R., & Good, G. E. (1997). Men in psychotherapy: An investigation of alexithymia, intimacy, and masculine gender roles. *Psychotherapy, 24*, 160–170.

Fletcher, R. (2011). *The Dad Factor: How Father-Baby Bonding Helps a Child for Life*. Sydney: Finch Publishing.

Gawlik, S., Müller, M., Hoffmann, L., Dienes, A., Wallwiener, M., Sohn, C., . . . Reck, C. (2014). Prevalence of paternal perinatal depressiveness and its link to partnership satisfaction and birth concerns. *Archives of Women's Mental Health, 17*, 49–56.

Giallo, R., Cooklin, A., Wade, C., D'Esposito, F., & Nicholson, J. M. (2014). *Fathers' Postnatal Mental Health and Child Wellbeing at Aged Five: The Mediating Role of Parental Self-Efficacy and Parenting Behaviour*. Paper presented at the LSAC & LSIC Research Conference, Melbourne.

Goldberg, W. (2014). *Father Time: The Social Clock and the Timing of Fatherhood*. London: Palgrave Macmillan.

Goodman, J. (2004). Paternal postpartum depression, its relationship to maternal postpartum depression, and implications for family health. *Journal of Advanced Nursing, 45*(1), 26–35.

Grossmann, K., Grossmann, K. E., Fremmer-Bombik, E., Kindler, H., Scheuerer-Englisch, H., & Zimmerman, P. (2002). The uniqueness of the child-father attachment relationship: Fathers' sensitive and challenging play as a pivotal variable in a 16-year longitudinal study. *Social Development, 11*, 307–331.

Harris, K. M., Furstenberg, F. F., & Marmer, K. J. (1998). Paternal involvement with adolescents in intact families: The influence of fathers over the life course. *Demography, 35*(2), 201–216.

Heim, C., Newport, D. J., Heit, S., Graham, Y. P., Wilcox, M., Bonsall, R., . . . Nemeroff, C. B. (2000). Pituitary-adrenal and autonomic responses to stress in women after sexual and physical abuse in childhood. *Journal of the American Medical Association, 284*, 592–597.

Hochschild, A. R. (1994). *Understanding the Future of Fatherhood: The "Daddy Hierarchy" and Beyond*. WORC Paper. Tillburg.

Hudson, B. D., Elek, S. M., & Fleck, M. O. (2001). First-time mothers' and fathers' transition to parenthood: Infant care self-efficacy, parenting satisfaction, and infant sex. *Issues in Comprehensive Pediatric Nursing, 24*(1), 31–43.

Hynan, M. T., Mounts, K. O., & Vanderbilt, L. D. (2013). Screening parents of high-risk infants for emotional distress: Rationale and recommendations. *Journal of Perinatology, 33*, 748–753.

Kessler, R. C., Berglund, P., Demler, O., Jin, R., Koretz, D., Merikangas, K. R., . . . Wang, P. S. (2003). The epidemiology of major depressive disorder: Results from the national

Comorbidity Survey Replication (NCS-R). *Journal of American Medical Association, 289,* 3095–3105.
Kim, P., & Swain, J. E. (2007). Sad dads: Paternal postpartum depression. *Psychiatry (Edgmont), 4,* 35–47.
Lamb, M. E. (1995). The changing role of fathers. In J. L. Shapiro, M. J. Diamond, & M. Greenberg (Eds.), *Becoming a Father* (pp. 18–35). New York: Springer.
Lamb, M. E. (Ed.) (2010). *The Role of the Father in Child Development* (5th ed.). Hoboken, NJ: Wiley.
Lamb, M. E., Pleck, J. H., Charnov, E. L., & Levine, J. A. (1987). A biosocial perspective on paternal behavior and involvement. In B. Lancaster, J. Altaman, A. Rossi, & R. L. Sherrod (Eds.), *Parenting Across the Life Span: Biosocial Perspectives* (pp. 11–42). New York: Academic Press.
Lara, M. A., Navarro, C., & Navarrete, L. (2010). Outcome results of a psycho-educational intervention in pregnancy to prevent PPD: A randomized control trial. *Journal of Affective Disorders, 122,* 109–117.
Levant, R. F. (1995). Toward the reconstruction of masculinity. In R. F. Levant & W. S. Pollack (Eds.), *The New Psychology of Men* (pp. 229–251). New York: Basic Books.
Matthey, S., Barnett, B., Howie, P., & Kavanagh, D. J. (2003). Diagnosing postpartum depression in mothers and fathers: Whatever happened to anxiety? *Journal of Affective Disorders, 74,* 139–147.
Matthey, S., Barnett, B., Kavanagh, D. J., & Howie, P. (2001). Validation of the Edinburgh Postnatal Depression Scale for men, and comparison of item endorsement with their partners. *Journal of Affective Disorders, 64,* 174–184.
McBride, B. A., Brown, G. L., Bost, K. K., Shin, N., Vaughn, B., & Korth, B. (2005). Paternal identity, maternal gatekeeping, and father involvement. *Family Relations, 54,* 360–372.
McKelley, R. A., & Rochlen, A. B. (2015). Furthering fathering: What we know and what we need to know. In Y. J. Wong & S. R. Wester (Eds.), *APA Handbook of Men and Masulinities* (pp. 525–549). Washington, DC: American Psychological Association.
Miller, M. (2012). Boot Camp for New Dads: Report on Workshop Surveys. Maggie Miller Consulting. (Accessed on December 17, 2015). Retrieved from http://www.bootcampfornewdads.org/validating-research
Murdock, K. W. (2013). An examination of parental self-efficacy among mothers and fathers. *Psychology of Men & Masculinity, 14*(3), 314–343. doi: 10.1037/a0027009
Musser, K. A., Ahmed, A. H., Foli, K. J., & Coddington, J. A. (2013). Paternal postpartum depression: What health care providers should know. *Journal of Pediatric Health Care, 27*(6), 479–485.
Occupational Outlook Handbook. (2015). U.S. Department of Labor, Bureau of Labor Statistics 2014. Retrieved from http://www.bls.gov/ooh/
O'Neil, J. M. (1990). Assessing men's gender role conflict. In D. Moore & F. Leafgren (Eds.), *Problem Solving Strategies and Interventions for Men in Conflict* (pp. 23–38). Alexandria, VA: American Counseling Association.
Panter-Brick, C., Burgess, A., Eggerman, M., McAllister, F., Pruett, K., & Leckman, J. F. (2014). Practitioner review: Engaging fathers—recommendations for a game change in parenting interventions based on a systematic review of the global evidence. *Journal of Child Psychology and Psychiatry, 11,* 1187–1212.
Paquette, D. (2004). Theorizing the father-child relationship: Mechanisms and developmental outcomes. *Human Development, 47,* 193–219.

Parke, R. (1996). *Fatherhood.* Cambridge, MA: Harvard University Press.
Patulny, R. (2011). *The Social Penalty of Work/Family Balance: Comparing Australian Men and Women's Social Contact with Ex Household Friends and Family.* Paper presented at the Australian Sociological Association Conference, Newcastle, England.
Paulson, F. J., & Bazemore, S. D. (2010). Prenatal and postpartum depression in fathers and its association with maternal depression: A meta-analysis. *Journal of the American Medical Association, 303,* 1961–1969.
Paulson, F. J., Dauber, S. E., & Leiferman, J. A. (2006). Individual and combined effects of maternal and paternal depression on parenting behavior. *Pediatrics, 118,* 659–668.
Pinheiro, K. A. T., Pinheiro, R. T., da Silva, A. R., da Cunha Coelho, F. M., de Ávila Quevedo, L., . . . Oses, J. P. (2011). Chronicity and severity of maternal postpartum depression and infant sleep disorders: A population-based cohort study in southern Brazil. *Infant Behavior and Development, 34,* 371–373.
Pleck, J. H. (1976). The male sex role: Definitions, problems, and sources of change. *Journal of Social Issues, 32,* 155–164.
Pleck, J. H. (2010). Paternal involvement: Revised conceptualization and theoretical linkages with child outcomes. In M. E. Lamb (Ed.), *The Role of the Father in Child Development* (5th ed., pp. 67–107). New York: Wiley.
Quinn, R. P., & Staines, G. L. (1979). *The 1977 Quality of Employment Survey.* Ann Arbor: University of Michigan.
Rabinowitz, F. E. L., & Cochran, S. V. (2008). Men and therapy: A case of masked male depression. *Clinical Case Studies, 7,* 575–591.
Radloff, L. S. (1977). The CES-D scale a self-report depression scale for research in the general population. *Applied Psychological Measurement, 1,* 385–401.
Ramchandani, P. G., Psychogiou, L., Vlachos, H., Les, J., Sethna, V., Netsi, E., & Lodder, A. (2011). Paternal depression: An examination of its links with father, child and family functioning in the postnatal period. *Depression and Anxiety, 28,* 471–477.
Ramchandani, P. G., Stein, A., Evans, J., & O'Connor, T. G. (2005). Paternal depression in the postnatal period and child development: A prospective population study. *Lancet, 365,* 2201–2205.
Rosenberg, J., & Wilcox, W. B. (2006). *The Importance of Fathers in the Healthy Development of Children: Fathers and Their Impact on Children's Well-Being.* U.S. Children's Bureau, Office on Child Abuse and Neglect. Retrieved from https://childwelfare.gov/pubPDFs/fatherhood.pdf
Roubinov, D. S., Luecken, L. J., Crnic, K. A., & Gonzales, N. A. (2014). Postnatal depression in Mexican American fathers: Demographic, cultural, and familial predictors. *Journal of Affective Disorders, 152,* 360–368.
Sanders, M. R. (1999). Triple P-Positive parenting program: Towards an empirically validated multilevel parenting and family support strategy for the prevention of behavior and emotional problems in children. *Clinical Child and Family Psychology Review, 22,* 71–90.
Sevigny, P. R., & Loutzenhiser, L. L. (2010). Predictors of parenting self-efficacy in mothers and fathers of toddlers. *Child: Care, Health and Development, 36,* 179–189.
Sheng, X., Le, H. N., & Perry, D. (2010). Perceived satisfaction with social support and depressive symptoms in perinatal Latinas. *Journal of Transcultural Nursing, 21,* 35–44.
Silverstein, L. B., Auerbach, C. F., & Levant, R. F. (2002). Contemporary fathers reconstructing masculinity: Clinical implications of gender role strain. *Professional Psychology: Research and Practice, 33*(4), 361–369.

Spector, A. Z. (2006). Fatherhood and depression: A review of risks, effects, and clinical application. *Issues in Mental Health Nursing, 27*, 8.

Storey, A. E., Walsh, C. J., Quinton, R. L., & Wynne-Edwards, K. E. (2000). Hormonal correlates of paternal responsiveness in new and expectant fathers. *Evolution and Human Behavior, 21*, 79–95.

Taylor, G. (1984). Alexithymia: Concept, measurement, and implications for treatment. *American Journal of Psychiatry, 141*, 725–732.

Twenge, J. M., Campbell, W. K., & Foster, C. A. (2003). Parenthood and marital satisfaction: A meta-analytic review. *Journal of Marriage and Family, 65*, 574–583.

Vogel, D. L., Wester, S. R., Hammer, J. H., & Downing-Matibag, T. M. (2014). Referring men to seek help: The influence of gender role conflict and stigma. *Psychology of Men & Masculinity, 15*, 60–67.

Waller, M. (2012). Cooperation, conflict, or disengagement? Coparenting styles and father involvement in fragile families. *Family Process, 51*(3), 325–342. doi: 10.1111/j.1545-5300.2012.01403.x

Wee, K. Y., Skouteris, H., Pier, C., Richardson, B., & Milgrom, J. (2011). Correlates of ante- and postnatal depression in fathers: A systematic review. *Journal of Affective Disorders, 130*, 358–377.

Yeung, W. J., Duncan, G. J., & Hill, M. S. (2000). Putting fathers back in the picture: Parental activities and children's adult outcomes. *Marriage and Family Review, 29*, 97–113.

Part II

Military Service and Perinatal Mental Health

Chapter 5

Introduction to Military Service and the Military Family

Melinda A. Thiam and Karen L. Weis

Introduction to Military Service

The military is a large organization, composed of five major divisions: U.S. Army, U.S. Air Force, U.S. Navy, U.S. Marines and U.S. Coast Guard. According to the demographic report in 2012, there are approximately 3.6 million service members serving within the total force, including Active duty, Reserve and National Guard service members. All military services are divided into officer and enlisted corps. Approximately 83.6% of the force is enlisted compared to the 16.4% of officers (Defense [DoD], 2013). Most military members have a minimum of a high school diploma and come from diverse backgrounds (Kane, 2005; McCrary, 2006).

Ever since the draft was discontinued post-Vietnam War in 1973, the American military has remained an all-volunteer force (Kane, 2005). Service members represent a diverse population in nearly every demographic category and geographic region across United States (Hamaoka et al., 2014). Thirty percent of active duty members identify themselves as ethnic minorities (Hamaoka et al., 2014)

Becoming a Service Member

Each service website has regulations governing who is eligible to join the service (Cardona & Ritchie, 2006). Troops are initially recruited dependent on the service specific requirements. In most cases, an individual must be 18 years old and have high school diploma, although sometimes a GED is accepted. Potential recruits undergo screening at a Military Entrance Processing Center and must take the Armed Services Vocational Aptitude Test (ASVAB) (Hamaoka et al., 2014). If applicants obtain the service specific score on ASVAB and meet rigorous medical and mental health standards, the recruit will enlist and subsequently go to service specific basic training. Basic training is meant to introduce recruits to the rigors of military life in physical, mental and emotional aspects. Basic training focuses on group cohesion, reduces individualism and builds a team mentality. This sense of teamwork and loyalty to the group identity creates a distinct community (Cox et al., 2006). After basic

Table 5.1 Introduction to Military Services

Service (Service Member)	*Purpose*	*Initial School*
Army *(Soldier)*	Largest force, specializes in ground defense (McCrary, 2006). Motto: "Army strong"; seven core values: loyalty, duty, respect, selfless service, honor, integrity and personal courage	Basic combat training—10 weeks at one of four training bases: Ft. Jackson, Ft. Leonardwood, Ft. Sill and Ft. Benning.
Air Force *(Airman)*	Mission to "fly, fight and win . . . in air, space and cyberspace"	Basic military training at Lackland Air Force Base, San Antonio, TX, for 8 ½ weeks followed by technical training
Navy *(Sailor)*	Sea/maritime defense and premier naval power—no official motto, "Non sibi sed patriae" ("Not self but country")	Boot camp at Great Lakes (7 weeks); followed by specialty training or "A school"
Coast Guard *(Sailor)*	Not technically Department of Defense; operates under Department of Homeland Security to protect nation's maritime interests; "Semper paratus" or "Always ready"	Basic training (8 weeks), either assigned an "A school" or receives a first duty station
Marines *(Marine)*	Expeditionary force in readiness; supports ground, aviation and amphibious operations trained to respond aggressively in times of crisis; "First to the fight"	Recruit training (12 weeks) Paris Island, SC

training, a recruit attends advanced training, which is where an individual learns how to do his or her job in the military. During initial entry training, recruits are in a restricted environment and typically reside in same barracks/living quarters. For recruits who are married, this is their first experience of separation from their spouse and family (see Table 5.1).

Military Lifestyle and Culture

Reasons for Joining

The military by nature has its own unique culture, language and customs. These customs are often unique to the specific military service. Since the 1970s, the military has been an all-volunteer force, and more service members have families (Hamaoka et al., 2014). Many individuals join to follow family tradition (Blue Star Families, 2015). Others may join because of their sense of patriotism and idealistic values of serving their countries. Finally, some individuals will join the military because they see it as a chance to transition into adulthood due to the military culture emphasis on personal responsibility, health, constant training, self-improvement and civic engagement (Kelty, Kleykamp, & Segal, 2010).

Gender and Military Service

Military service has traditionally been seen as a male role, but since establishment of an all-volunteer force in 1972, equal opportunity has allowed women to have more opportunities in the military services (Kelty et al., 2010). Today, female service members make up 14 % of the enlisted population (compared to 2% in 1973) and 16% of the officers (compared to 4% in 1973) and are around 15% of the total force (Department of Defense, 2014). Only 46% of active duty women are married, compared to 58% of active duty men (Patten & Parker, 2009). Almost half of married active duty women are married to a fellow service member compared to 7% of military men and are more likely to be single parents—12% are single moms compared to 4% single dads (Patten & Parker, 2009).

Military Benefits

After joining the military, an individual has job security, health benefits, and a secure salary. Military pay is based off the Department of Defense pay scale, and provides a base salary based on rank and time in service (Hamaoka et al., 2014). Single, junior enlisted members are provided living quarters, and there is usually base housing available if desired. Services members living off base receive Basic Allowance for Housing (BAH) to help offset cost of mortgage/rent and Basic Allowance Sustenance (BAS) to offset cost of food (Hamaoaka et al., 2014). The military provides universal health care for active duty troops and families through TRICARE as well as subsidized dental care. Military educational benefits are based from the Montgomery GI Bill. The GI Bill can fund education and provide an individual with college education while concurrently serving on active duty (Hamaoka et al., 2014).

The Military Family

The demands of the military lifestyle create unique challenges for the military family. The military family makes up approximately 1% of the American population, and 70% of these families live in civilian communities. Over half of all service members are married, and 43% of service members are parents, with an estimated 2 million children in military families (DoD, 2014). Approximately 36 % of married military members are parents, while 7% of military members are single parents (DoD, 2014). Military service members are more likely to be married at a younger age, and have children at home than civilian counterparts in this category (Blue Star Families, 2015). Military families frequently marry young. The average age of an active duty service member at the birth of first child is 25 years old. Within the total military force, over 43% of service members are parents, with 37.5% of these children under age 5. The marital status of officers is 65.5% compared to 53.3% of married enlisted service members. While the percentage of children under 5 in total force is 37.5%, when restricted to Active duty force, this age is 42.4% (DoD, Nov 2013).

Marriage and the Military

Today's volunteer military force is older, more career oriented and more family oriented. Service members may enter single, but then marry once in active service (Kelty et al., 2010). Military personnel are more likely to be married in comparison to civilian counterparts, and the mean age of the women at the birth of their first child is 1.5 years younger for military women compared to civilian women (Kelty et al., 2010).

The Military Spouse

Military spouses are said to hold a "keystone role" in establishing a healthy home environment (Joseph, 2014). Military spouses have to assimilate into the military just as their active duty partner, and the whole family "serves" in military. Military spouses are relied upon to become the primary caregiver, make occupational sacrifices, deal with financial concerns independently, organize relocations and cope with the lack of social support (Joseph, 2014). Most military spouses are female, and only 9% of civilian spouses are male (Jebo, 2005). The support structures within the military system traditionally assume that a military spouse is female; furthermore, both family readiness groups and spousal support groups predominantly tailor to female spouses (Jebo, 2005). The civilian male spouse may feel awkward in this environment, as he may not feel included in the spouses group (predominately women), and feel uncomfortable/unsupported on the military base. Military officer spouses may be expected to engage in volunteer services at the family readiness group (FRG), youth activities and social events to support her husband's unit (Kelty et al., 2010). Military spouses are also expected to support the active duty member's career, even if this means lost employment and educational opportunities for themselves (Kelty et al., 2010).

The Military Child

The military child has gained increasing attention over the past years, as awareness has been raised regarding the impact of deployment on children's health and well-being. Military children are faced with frequent separation from their mothers or fathers. In dual-military families, this can mean children stay with extended family/childcare providers for long periods of time (Murphey, Darling-Churchhill, & Chrisler, 2011). The Blue Star Families (BSF) study found that military children under the age of 10 have spent 20% of their lives separated from at least one of their parents (Blue Star Families, 2015). Even when parents are not deployed, many have such demanding jobs in the current environment that they are essentially never home. Children may feel rejected by the absent service member parent and not able to connect with the distressed caregiver at home (McFarlane, 2009).

Impact of Military Life on Families

Military lifestyle is dynamic (regardless of deployment) and requires families to be adaptable, resilient and patient in an environment characterized by uncertainty (Blue Star Families, 2015). For example, military families are exposed to stressors similar to civilian families. They have financial goals that require dual incomes, concerns about pay and benefits, concerns about childcare and education as well as a desire to develop/foster relationships in the community (Blue Star Families, 2015). Stressors unique to military lifestyle include deployment, frequent moves and changes in duty location, geographical separation for reasons related to deployment as well as other circumstances, unique spouse employment challenges, unique child and spouse education (Blue Star Families, 2015).

Blue Star Families (BSF) is a large and fast growing nonprofit organization focused on supporting the military family that works with other organizations to improve awareness of challenges and strengths of military families (Blue Star Families, 2015). The BSF organization annually creates a comprehensive report that identifies the key aspects of military life to target resources, services and programs that support the sustainability of the all-volunteer force (Blue Star Families, 2015). With the congressionally mandated military draw-down, the various branches of the military are being asked to do more with less, which continues to lead to prolonged periods of geographical separation for prolonged periods of time (Blue Star Families, 2015).

Military families are central to service member recruitment, retention and readiness. Issues that impact military families thus impacts troop readiness. The following sections will discuss the areas that hold the most prevalent challenges for military families (Blue Star Families, 2015).

Frequent Relocation and Geographic Separation

Military service requires a mobile lifestyle with frequent military moves within the United States and around the world. Service members are usually stationed at their duty station for 2–3 years at a time, which then requires geographical location for an entire family. The BSF survey reported that military families moved 7 times more than civilian families (Blue Star Families, 2015). In addition to relocation, military families frequently face long periods of separation. Military service members are assigned to a specific permanent duty station, but then have to undergo field training, service and career school, temporary duties in other areas as well as deployment. In 2015, BSF found 30% of Active duty service members were separated from familes for an addition 6–12 months unrelated to deployment (Blue Star Families, 2015). In addition to military assignments/duties that require separation, there are instances where military families are voluntarily living apart for various reason called "geo-baching" usually as a means to create stability for their families (Blue Star Families, 2014, 2015). The three most common reasons for intentional geographic separation include: very short duty assignments that are not long enough to warrant relocating (34%), separation due to spouse's career (34%) and to support/stabilize their children's education (27%) (Blue Star Families, 2015). Additional reasons for such separations include financial reasons/cost of living concerns (23%) as well as the inability to sell a home (13%) (Blue Star Families, 2015).

Financial and Economic Challenges

Approximately 85% of military service members joined for financial security, but due to current economic concerns, financial uncertainty is one of the top stressors for military families (Blue Star Families, 2015). The top financial concerns are related to four main issues: uncertainty in military life (42%), spouse employment concerns (40%), saving for retirement (39%) and frequent moves and changes in duty station (32%) (Blue Star Families, 2015). In particular, frequent moves and relocations add to financial constraints. BSF found that 73% of military families identified military moves as one of the main unexpected expenses that result from military service (Blue Star Families, 2015). Financial problems can lead to significant distress. Families also have challenges related to buying/selling homes. When military families buy a home, they often take a financial loss when they usually inevitably sell under a short timeline (Blue Star Families, 2015). In the BSF survey, 10% of home owners were "upside down" on mortgages" (Blue Star Families, 2015). Although housing is available on base, many military families prefer to live off base due to concerns for lack of privacy, on base housing was too small or the wait list too long (Blue Star Families, 2015; MacDermid et al., 2004)

Military service members may experience financial hardship (Blue Star Families, 2015). Financial hardship is impacted by the service member's rank, spouse employment, and cost of living in the area. For a junior enlisted service member with a large family, the combined costs of expenses can lead to difficulty balancing a budget. BSF found that 20% of active duty families had over $10,000 in credit card debt, 8% had over $20,000 in credit card debt and 3% held nine or more credit cards (Blue Star Families, 2015). Additionally, despite all the benefits and entitlements given to military families, there are military families that still fall below the federal poverty level and are eligible for food stamps. A family is eligible for food stamps if the monthly income is below 130% of Federal Poverty Level, which can make an E-4 who is a sole provider with four children eligible for up to $200/month (Hosek & MacDermid-Wadsworth, 2013; MacDermid et al., 2004). Alarmingly, the BSF survery reported that 26% of families had particpated in Women, Infants and Children (WIC), 7% had a household member who faced food insecurity and 6% sought emergency food assitance (Blue Star Families, 2015).

Current Economic Challenges: Reduction in Force

Beginning in 2011, after a decade of war, the economic and political factors changed: instead of continuing to build up the military, the military was mandated to begin restructuring and downsizing its force (Feickert, 2014). In January 2012, it was noted that 90,000 soldiers were deployed in support of operations and another 96,000 soldiers were forward-stationed overseas in nearly 150 countries. Despite this number, Congress mandated that the Army downsize from a peak of 570,000 soldiers to 490,000 soldiers (Feickert, 2014). This number continues to be decreased. In 2013, the Army had to accelerate downsizing, which led to a significant reduction of forces and involuntary separation of mid-level officers and prevention of mid-level non-commissioned officers from promotion, thus leading to forced retirement (Feickert, 2014). Similar downsizing is occurring across all the services, with increased mandatory separations without an option of retirement. However, despite the drawdown in the Middle East compared to years between 2003–2010, the mission of the military has continued, and units have to continue to do more missions with less (Moakler, 2014). Previously, individuals have been interested in the military due to benefits—this includes free health care, access to services such as commissaries (reduced fee grocery stores), a basic allowance for housing (BAH) and a guaranteed salary. Now, families are faced with economic uncertainties such as whether they will be selected for involuntary retirement, lower pay raises, commissary cuts, reduced BAH and less medical coverage (Moakler, 2014).

Spouse Employment

Military service members are expected to be available 24-7 and at any time can be called away to work, sent to school or deployed. Given such, military spouses can have challenges finding employment, just to pick up and have to leave again in 2–3 years. In the BSF survey, 75% of active duty spouses indicated that their military affiliation has a negative impact on their ability to pursue a career (Blue Star Families, 2015). Military spouses frequently experience a loss of control over their career due to frequent, unexpected, unwanted or unanticipated moves, or feel pressure to prioritized their children's needs or their service members career over their own (Blue Star Families, 2015). Research on military families has also shown that when military spouses are employed, they are employed at lower rates, work fewer hours, and for less pay than their civilian counterparts with comparable education, experience, age and marital status (Blue Star Families, 2015; Maury & Stone, 2014). One of the top factors that lead to military spouse unemployment includes the negative impact of military lifestyle (Blue Star Families, 2015). Many factors that fall under negative impact of military lifestyle include significant household duties (especially if spouse is deployed), childcare duties and unpredictable service member work schedule that frequently prevent active duty members from reliably supporting family childcare needs (Blue Star Families, 2015). Other factors include poor job market alignment and perceived differential treatment from employers or potential employers (Blue Star Families, 2015).

Military Child and Spouse Education

As mentioned above, over 43% of service members are parents (DoD, 2014). Frequent moves are not only disruptive for the service member and spouse; they are also disruptive for children. According to the Military Interstate Children's Compact Commission, the average military child will attend six to nine different schools in their lives, with at least two transitions in high school (Blue Star Families, 2015; Johnson, Knauss, Faran, & Ban, 2014). One study found that the average military child moved six to nine times before high school. Changing school systems can be extremely challenging for both children and parents (Blue Star Families, 2015). When parents inevitably move between states, the education rules for graduation vary by state. Changing schools can introduce various concerns such as curriculum requirements, services and extracurricular activities that are rarely consistent from one school district to the next (Blue Star Families). Many public schools have no means of identifying military children, and many teachers are unaware when they have military children in their classrooms. In the Blue Star Families survey, 60% of respondents did not feel that their school created opportunities to celebrate and include the military (Blue Star Families, 2015). Nowadays, public schools located close to military bases have a designated school liaison, and military base child and youth services also have a designated school representative.

Childcare Challenges

Like many families with small children, military families often struggle with finding high quality yet affordable childcare (Blue Star Families, 2015). For dual active duty families, dual career families or active duty single parents, families struggle with additional challenges of finding care that works around military schedules. Depending on the job and work factors, military service members may have to work 24-hour shifts, extended hours and weekend duty shifts (Blue Star Families, 2015). In certain duty stations, such as training bases, certain jobs such as Drill Sergeant, are stateside/nondeployable assignments, but require very long hours, frequently from 0400 (4:00 am) in morning until 2100 (9:00 pm) at night. In the military, there are Child Developmental Centers (CDC) that offer care for children from 6 weeks to 12 years old (Blue Star Families, 2015). The ability to find quality childcare is critical. For single active duty service members or dual-military, lack of adequate childcare can lead to separation from military service. Active duty women married to civilian spouses may have significant difficulty finding childcare on base because the system is focused on the male being the working spouse, which often places active duty women last on the list for military childcare.

Deployment

In the past 12 years, over 2 million military service members have served in Operation Enduring Freedom, Operation Iraqi Freedom and Operation New Dawn with over 3.3 million deployments (Chandra et al., 2010). Stresses of combat exposure create unique mental health challenges in both service members and families. These particular challenges include extended separations (sometimes up to 17 months at a time), frequent deployments, and compromised parenting due to traumatic exposure (in service member or transmitted second-hand to family members). Deployment frequency has increased with subsequent deployments sometimes only 9–12 months apart. Military deployments may come with very little advance notice, and some deployments (particularly in Special Forces and specialized units) are unexpected and locations cannot be communicated to family members. In these cases, the family has limited to no communication during the deployment or operation, and a date of return is unknown. As the war died down over the past 2 years, the military force has entered into a significant drawdown, and military members/families are rapidly transitioning out of the military and into civilian communities, which leads to additional challenges as military veterans and their families struggle with the untreated illnesses resulting from military service (Clervil, Grandin, & Greendlinger, 2010).

Younger children still have the developmental phenomena called "magical thinking" where they will assume their parents' behavior is directly related to something they did or did not do. Parents who are stressed or exposed to trauma have higher rates of child maltreatment. Particularly, a parent returning with Post Traumatic Stress Disorder (PTSD) can affect the child due to the effects of PTSD on parenting (de Burgh, White, Fear & Iversen, 2011).

Mental injuries affect not just the service member but the entire family. In particular, effects of PTSD in service members reverberate throughout the family. PTSD is marked by emotional avoidance and disengagement of the affected individual (Cozza, Chun, & Polo, 2014). A parent with PTSD returning from combat may be reluctant to engage with his or her children, may remain emotionally avoidant or may be easily irritated. Some parents may struggle to engage with their children, particularly if part of the combat trauma involved the death of other children; hugging or interacting with their child may trigger memories of combat. Their hyper-arousal symptoms can lead a parent to poorly tolerate frequent childhood behaviors such as arguing, engaging in physical play or participating in family routines.

Behavioral Health Challenges

In addition to stressors for family members, active duty service members are reporting higher levels of mental health issues (Blue Star Families, 2015). Despite the national attention on occurrence of depression or PTSD in service members, many studies have found that only 53% of returning troops who meet criteria for PTSD or major depression sought help in the last year (Blue Star Families, 2015). Even though these numbers indicate active duty service member and family member reluctance to seek help, over 30% of survey respondents reported receiving some form of mental health counseling—this was often off post and more often relied on civilian network providers (Blue Star Families, 2014, 2015). Other studies confirm that rates of depression and anxiety increase when an active duty service member is deployed (Shannon et al., 2007; Mansfield et al., 2010; Verdeli et al., 2011).

Behavioral Health Resonates through Families

There is a concept of "stress spillover" where external stressors (such as employment or financial concerns) adversely affect the marriage relationship and subsequently spillover into parent–child relationships (Paley, Lester, & Mogil, 2013). Children can usually recognize marital conflict even if parents feel that it is "hidden." Young children are particularly attuned to parent nonverbal behaviors and may perceive distress in a parent even before a parent may recognize such feelings (McFarlane, 2009). Exposure to parental conflict has significant consequences to children in many areas and has been linked to increased internalizing/externalizing behaviors, increased emotional insecurity and poorer academic functioning (Park, 2011; Riggs & Riggs, 2011).

Summary

President Obama has made the care and support of military families a top national security policy priority (Biden, 2011) because the well-being of military families directly affects troop readiness. In the words of President Obama,

> Let me be clear, stronger military families will strengthen the fabric of America. By spotlighting their devotion, to service, internal resilience, and patriotism, all Americans will have examples to emulate. I will ensure the commitment, partnerships, and resources endure well after the guns are silenced and our service members come home.
>
> (Biden, 2011)

This chapter has described a basic introduction to military service, makeup of the military family and challenges innate to military families. From this foundation, the next chapter will explore the perinatal mental health challenges in military families.

References

Biden, J. (January 24, 2011). *Strengthening Our Military Families: Meeting America's Committment* [Press Release].

Blue Star Families. (2014). Military Family Life Survey: Comprehensive Report. Department of Research and Policy. Retrieved from: https://www.bluestarfam.org/resources/military-family-lifestyle-survey

Blue Star Families. (2015). Military Family Lifestyle Survey: Comprehensive Report. Department of Research and Policy. Retrieved from https://www.bluestarfam.org/resources/military-family-lifestyle-survey

Cardona, R., & Ritchie, E. (2006). Psychological screening of recruits prior to accession in the US military. In Martha Lenhart, Dave Lunsbury, Robert North (Eds.), *Recruit Medicine*. Fort Sam Houston, TX: Office of the Surgeon General, at TMM Publications. The Borden Institute. Walter Reed Army Medical Center, Washington, D.C, 20307. Retrieved from http://www.cs.amedd.army.mil/borden/portal

Chandra, A., Lara-Cinisomo, S., Jaycox, L., Tanielian, T., Burns, R., Ruder, T., & Han, B. (2010). Children on the homefront: The experience of children from military families. *Pediatrics, 125*, 16–25.

Clervil, R., Grandin, M., & Greendlinger, R. (2010). Understanding the Experience of Military Familes and Their Returning War Fighters. Retrieved from http://montgomery.md.networkofcare.org/content/pdf/100.pdf

Cox, A., Edison, D., Stewart, R., Dorson, C., & Ritchie, E. (2006). Management of recruit suicide. In Martha Lenhart, Dave Lunsbury, Robert North (Eds.), *Recruit Medicine* [E-Reader Version]. Fort Sam Houston, TX: Office of the Surgeon General, Deparatment of the Army S Army Medical Department Center and School. Retrieved from http://www.cs.amedd.army.mil/borden/

Cozza, S., Chun, R., & Polo, J. (2005). Military families and children during operation Iraqi freedom. *Pscyhiatric Quarterly, 76*(4), 371–378.

de Burgh, H. T., White, C. J., Fear, N. T., & Iversen, A. C. (2011). The impact of deployment to Iraq or Afghanistan on partners and wives of military personnel. *International Review Psychiatry, 23*(2), 192–200. doi:10.3109/09540261.2011.560144

Department of Defense. (2014). 2014 Demographics: Profile of Military Community. Office of the Deputy Assistant Secretary of Defense. Retrieved from http://www.militaryonesource.mil

Feickert, A. (2014). Army Drawdown and Restructuring: Background and Issues for Congress. Retrieved from https://www.fas.org/sgp/crs/natsec/R42493.pdf

Hamaoka, D., Bates, M., McCarrol, J., Brim, W., Lunasco, T., & Rhodes, J. (2014). Introduction to military service. In S. Cozza, M. Goldenberg, & R. Ursano (Eds.), *Caring for Military Service Members, Veterans, and their Families* [E-Reader Version]. Arlington, VA: American Psychiatric Publishing, Inc. Retrieved from http://dx.doi.org/10.1176/appi.books.9781585625161.sc01

Hosek, J., & MacDermid-Wadsworth, S. (2013). Economic conditions of military families. *The Future of Children, 23*(2), 41–59.

Jebo, Jennifer. (2005). An Untraditional Life: Male Spouses of Female Military Personnel. Dissertation submitted to Virgina Polytechnic Institute and State University, Blacksburg, VA.

Johnson, P., Knauss, L., Faran, M., & Ban, P. (2014). Military children & programs that meet their needs. In S. Cozza, M. Goldenberg, & R. Ursano (Eds.), *Care of Military Service Members, Veterans, and Their Families* [E-Reader Version]. Arlington, VA: American Psychiatric Publishing, Inc. Retrieved from http://dx.doi.org/10.1176/appi.books.9781585625161.sc03

Joseph, Cristina. (2014). Examining Chronic Stress in Spouses of Active Duty Military Members. Dissertation submitted for partial fulfillment of Master of Science in Nursing, School of Nursing, Rhode Island College. Paper 47. Retrieved from: http://digitalcommons.ric.edu/school_of_nursing/47

Kane, T. (2005). *Who Bears the Burden? Demographic Characteristics of U.S. Military Recruits before and after 9/11.* Washington, DC: The Heritage Foundation. Retrieved from http://www.heritage.org/research/reports/2005/11/who-bears-the-burden-demographic-characteristics-of-us-military-recruits-before-and-after-9-11

Kelty, R., Kleykamp, M., & Segal, D. (2010). The military and the transition to adulthood. *Future Child, 20*(1), 181–207.

MacDermid, S., Strauss, R., Robbins, N., Wenz, H., Chang, Y., Schwarz, R., . . . Kontos, S. (2004). *The Financial Landscape for Military Families of Young Children.* West Lafayette, IN: Military Family Research Institute, Purdue University. Retrieved from: https://www.mfri.purdue.edu/resources/public/reports/Financial%20Landscape%20of%20Families.pdf

Mansfield, A. J., Kaufman, J. S., Marshall, S. W., Gaynes, B. N., Morrissey, J. P., & Engel, C. C. (2010). Deployment and the use of mental health services among U.S. army wives. *New England Journal of Medicine, 362*(2), 101–109. doi:10.1056/NEJMoa0900177

Maury, R., & Stone, B. (2014). *Military Spouse Employment Report.* Institute for Veterans and Military Families under Military Officers Association of America. Syracuse University, NY. Retrieved from http://vets.syr.edu/wp-content/uploads/2014/02/MilitarySpouseEmploymentReport_2013.pdf

McCrary, James. (2006). Overview of recruiting and accessions. In Martha Lenhart, Dave Lunsbury, Robert North (Eds.), *Recruit Medicine.* Fort Sam Houston, TX: Office of the

Surgeon General, Deparatment of the Army S Army Medical Department Center and School. Retrieved from http://www.cs.amedd.army.mil/borden/portal

McFarlane, A. (2009). Military deployment: The impact on children and family adjustment and need for care. *Current Opinion in Psychiatry, 22*, 369–373.

Moakler, K. (2014). National Military Family Association leads discussion on transitioning families out of the military. National Military Family Association. Retrieved from http://www.militaryfamily.org/about us/press/2014/transitioning.html#sthash.XzTrsks1.dpuf

Murphey, D., Darling-Churchhill, K., & Chrisler, Alison. (2011). *The Well-Being of Young Children in Military Families: A Review and Recommendations for Further Study*. Washington, DC: Child Trends Publication #2011–21.

Paley, B., Lester, P., & Mogil, C. (2013). Family systems and ecological perspectives on the impact of deployment on military families. *Clinical Child and Family Psychological Review, 16*(3), 245–265. doi: 10.1007/s10567-013-0138-y. Retrieved from https://www.ncbi.nlm.nih.gov/pubmed/23760926

Park, N. (2011). Military children and families strengths and challenges during peace and war. *American Psychologist, 66*(1), 65–72.

Patten, E., & Parker, K. (2009). Women in the U.S. Military: Growing Share, Distinctive Profile. *Report to the White House Councilon Women and Girls*. Department of Defense, September 1, 2009. Retrieved from www.pewsocialtrends.org

Riggs, S., & Riggs, D. (2011). Risk and resilience in military families experiencing deployment: The role of the family attachment network. *Journal of Family Psychology, 25*(5), 675–687.

Shannon, J., Johnson, C., Michelle, D., Sherman, C. C., Hoffman, J. S., James, L. C., . . . Riggs, D. (February 2007). *The Psychological Needs of U.S. Military Service Members and Their Families: A Preliminary Report*. The American Psychological Association. Retrieved from https://www.apa.org/about/policy/military-deployment-services.pdf

Verdeli, H., Baily, C., Vousoura, E., Belser, A., Manos, G., & Singla, D. (2011). The case for treating depression in military spouses. *Journal of Family Psychology, 25*(4), 488–496. doi:10.1037/a0024525

Chapter 6

Perinatal Mental Health in the Military

Melinda A. Thiam, Eric M. Flake, Kelly O. Elmore, Michael M. Dickman, and Kellie Haworth

Introduction

> "I am 37 weeks pregnant with my third baby and my husband is being deployed immediately after I deliver. I had postpartum depression with both my pregnancies, so I am very stressed and concerned now with knowing whom to talk to and go to since I am not familiar with this area or the base. I have a 2yr old & 3yr old at home currently, so I wasn't expecting to be on my own right away with a newborn, but I know that's how it is in the military. It is just very stressful preparing and the baby hasn't even come! Also knowing that my own potential deployment will be coming up shortly if not immediately when my husband gets back, and he won't even know our new baby, just a lot of stress."
>
> —Submitted to Postpartum Support International

Throughout this book, we have discussed how perinatal mental health is a dynamic mix of biological, socio-environmental and psychological factors that affect the expression of a disease. This chapter adds one more aspect to the paradigm: the environment of care via the Military Health System (MHS). This chapter will explore how military culture and the environment of care affect the biopsychosocial aspects of pregnancy as illustrated in Figure 6.1.

The Military Health Care System

Perinatal mental health is a form of interdisciplinary medicine. In the civilian environment, a collaboration of care can be challenging due to patients having differing availability and accessibility to quality health care, particularly specialty care. Each health care plan or health care system may have different types of treatment processes that create challenges accessing specialty care in the surrounding network. In contrast, military families are cared for by a single system: Military Health System (MHS). Military providers share a common mission to care for the service member and his/her family. Military

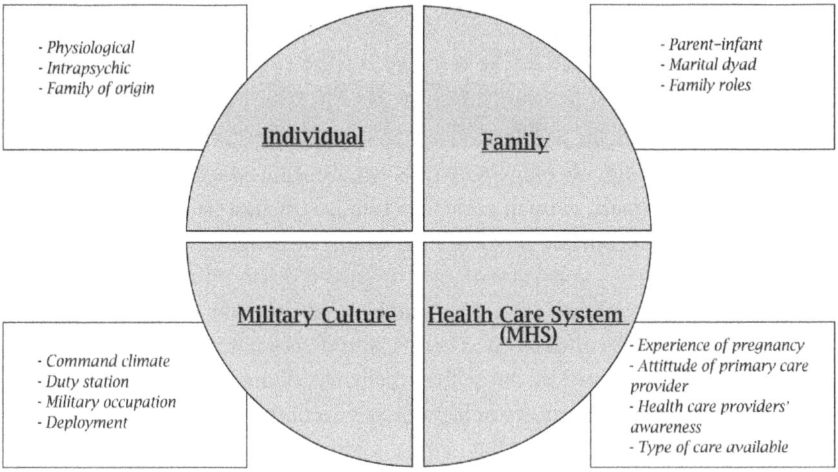

Figure 6.1 System Paradigms Impacting Perinatal Mental Health

providers are composed of Active Duty and /or Reserve providers, Department of Defense (DoD) contractor civilian providers, and Government Service (GS) civilian providers. Military primary care providers often work in close proximity with military specialty providers, or at least have the ability to consult through telehealth. The common language of military medicine and uniformity of the electronic health care record enables collaboration amongst primary care and specialists.

Military medicine has been a vital source of advancing the medical field in a variety of disciplines, and providers train to provide good medicine in austere environments, and, in addition to medical care in the combat environment, military providers have provided invaluable expertise during natural disasters or humanitarian missions. In 2006, military providers at a military treatment facility demonstrated their ability to provide excellent care in bad places during Hurricane Katrina. In 2006, military obstetrics and gynecology physicians made headlines after completing cesarean delivery by flashlight during the evacuation of Keesler Air Force Hospital (Allen, Flinn, & Moore, 2007; see Figure 6.2).

Military Medicine has the potential to develop multi-specialty programs to assess, diagnosis and treat perinatal mental health disorders. Different specialties that can contribute to such a program include obstetric care by certified nurse midwives, women's health nurse practitioners, obstetrician-gynecologists (OBGYN), and family medicine providers; pediatric care provided by pediatric nurse practitioners and physicians as well as family medicine physicians, nurse practitioners and physician assistants. Internal medicine and family

Caesarian by Flashlight?

The obstetrics and gynecology (OB/GYN) flight at Keeslaer Medical Center sheltered 36 pregnant women and their families during Hurricane Katrina to ensure that appropriate medical care would be available. Ironically, the hospital's emergency generators were destroyed during the 30-foot storm surge, while one woman with a previous cesarean section went into active labor. She ultimately underwent a cesarean delivery using battery-operated flashlights for illumination. After the storm, the damage to the hospital was so extensive as to require aeromedical evacuation of the pregnant patients and their families. (Allen, Flinn, & Moore, 2007)

Figure 6.2 Cesarean by Flashlight

medicine may provide care to the mother before or after pregnancy. These primary care providers are her "first responders" that engage in assessment and screening during different periods dependent on specialty. As first responders, these practitioners will identify and discuss maternal concerns, diagnose and initiate behavioral health consults and medical treatments. Behavioral health care providers and community services provide behavior health treatment of various intensity, depending on access and availability of treatment.

Military Obstetricians and Family Medicine

In military health care, mothers usually receive their postpartum care from certified nurse midwives, women's health nurse practitioners, physicians trained in obstetrics and gynecology or family medicine providers (Thomas, Sleath, Jackson, West, & Gaynes, 2008). Obstetric care for civilian spouses and active duty mothers is usually provided at the nearest medical treatment facility. Military obstetrics, including physicians, midwives and obstetric nursing, are at the forefront of perinatal health in the military. Obstetric providers in the military health clinic have expertise in understanding the military family and military culture and are cognizant of significant military events such as deployment or duty challenges that face active duty or dependent women. In these settings, providers work closely with both pediatric providers and have access to behavioral health specialists. On smaller bases or more remote areas that do not have military treatment facilities or a medical center nearby, families may be deferred to a network provider. Although network providers provide appropriate obstetric care, providers are frequently not acquainted with the intricacies that come with military life such as understanding why a spouse cannot just "come home" for a deployment or take time away from operational training to accompany the spouse to appointments.

Military obstetrics has been at forefront of research on perinatal depression, especially as it relates to deployments. Military obstetrics has created different interventions such as group prenatal care, and has provided treatment interventions that will be further explored in Chapter 9.

Military Pediatricians

Military pediatricians have been at the forefront of caring for military children, especially over the last decade, and they continue to bring awareness to the needs of the military child. Active duty military pediatricians and civilian pediatric providers are specially equipped to know how different aspects of military culture influence the military family. Military pediatricians, both active duty, and civilians, are in the "front line" caring for U.S. military children and their families and play a critical role in identifying how well or poorly a child or family responds to major stressors such as deployment or parent mental health issues. *Military Pediatrics* has published on many different topics and studies that discuss the impact of deployment on children. Due to the recognition of the impact of military lifestyle on the military child, the American Academy of Pediatrics has strongly supported the needs of military pediatricians and military children.

Military Family Medicine

Military family medicine providers are clinicians who provide care for the entire military family. Similar to family medicine providers in the civilian environment, military family medicine clinicians provide "womb-to-tomb" medicine. Military medicine providers provide obstetric/prenatal care, assist with delivery, and provide early postpartum care for mothers. Family medicine providers also can provide for infant care. Because family medicine providers treat both the parent and the child, they may be one of the first to notice that a mother or father is struggling. Military family medicine providers can diagnosis and treat depressive disorders and often work closely with behavioral health professionals.

Military family medicine providers are well acquainted with "good medicine in bad places," especially in their care of the active duty service member. Military family medicine providers are accustomed to military operational medicine and may work with military commands in many different aspects. Military family medicine providers have served at all levels ranging from clinical care to department chiefs, and several have reached the level of General Officer/Admiral, where they can influence military medicine on a larger scale.

Military Behavioral Health

Military behavioral health has been at the forefront of the treatment of mental disorders for the active duty service member. Military behavioral health has predominately focused on the active duty member and the increased rates of mental illness such as depression, PTSD, substance abuse, and TBI in active duty troops as well as the increasing suicide rate in active duty and veteran service members. Military behavioral health recognizes the influence of mental health in the military spouse and how a spouse's mental health affects the readiness of military service member.

Military child psychiatry, similar to military pediatrics, has focused on traumatic stress in children because of parent deployment and potential death or serious injury. Military child psychiatry has been leading the way in addressing the mental health care needs of military children and has led the way to develop collaborative treatment between primary care and behavioral health through the development of different integrated care programs such as Child and Family Behavioral Health Services. These programs will be discussed in more detail in Chapters 10 and 11.

Family Systems Perspective on Transition to Parenthood

The Military Spouse

> "I saw that you specialized in military families. I was wondering if you could provide me a resource in my area. I am no longer living near or on an installation. My husband had deployed to Afghanistan 9 days before the baby was born, so I went back home I really need help. I'm really sinking."

The Civilian Mother/Female Spouse

The female civilian spouse in the military family frequently experiences challenges of pregnancy and parenthood in a military family. Many of the challenges of the military spouse that were identified in the last chapter can negatively affect the pregnancy and postpartum periods. For instance, military spouses have to cope with challenges of pregnancy as well as challenges of military lifestyle (Schachman & Lindsey, 2013).

Despite the challenges of military life, military families are remarkably resilient and have some protective mechanisms in place. The same areas of military life that create challenges can also serve as a benefit due to cohesiveness of the military community and web of support within the military communities. The female civilian spouse often benefits from the formal and informal support that can have reciprocal and synergetic effects to support emotional and mental well-being. The shared history and experiences among military wives facilitate the spontaneous creation of informal, nontraditional support networks. Additional variables that have a protective influence on the lives of military wives include the development of self-reliant attitudes and behaviors (Schachman & Lindsey, 2013). Successful management of military stressors not only enhances the individual's sense of personal competence (Schachman & Lindsey, 2013), but also contributes to the development of a coping repertoire that can be used in future stressful situations, such as new motherhood (Schachman & Lindsey, 2013).

PREVALENCE

There is little research on the rates/prevalence of perinatal mood and anxiety disorders in the military civilian spouse. The Armed Forces Surveillance Study identified 8.2% rate of postpartum depression in military spouses; within this population there was 0.2% risk of suicidality (Do, Hu, Otto, & Rohrbeck, 2013). Research in military obstetrics and gynecology has identified increased prevalence of perinatal depression when an active duty service member deployed during his spouse's pregnancy (Danielson, 2010; Haas, Pazdernik, & Olsen, 2005; Robrecht, Millegan, Leventis, Crescitelli, & McLay, 2008; Smith, Munroe, Foglia, Nielsen, & Deering, 2010; Spooner, Rastle, & Elmore, 2012). Additionally, deployment during a spouse's pregnancy leads to higher risk of maternal complications such as preterm birth and low birthweight (Spieker, 2012; Tarney et al., 2015).

CONSIDERING MOTHERHOOD

Similar to the general population, military spouses often struggle with intentionally planning and timing their pregnancies. A military spouse may struggle with how to choose the best time to become pregnant, and she may feel that she has to plan her pregnancy around her spouse's career (Levine, Bukowinski, Sevick, Mehlhaff, & Conlin, 2015). If she becomes pregnant at an "inopportune time," this can lead to marriage challenges, and potentially affect her spouse's military readiness. If she does plan, the active duty service member may be deployed or must participate in an extended training at any time, and she may have to uproot/relocate during pregnancy.

ACCEPTANCE OF PREGNANCY AND COMMITMENT TO MATERNAL ROLE

Women frequently desire to involve their spouse in pre-pregnancy activities such as parenting classes, labor and delivery classes. However, due to the nature of military service, they must create a "backup plan" in the event their spouse is called away to duty during or after delivery. At larger medical centers, there are therapists embedded in obstetric clinics where a mother who is struggling with antepartum anxiety or depression may be assisted by a social worker who will help her with proper resources and referrals. In these cases, a case manager who works in close collaboration with the obstetric team may be able to assist with resources. Mothers may be referred to community resources to help with social support during pregnancy. In less common cases, during pregnancy, mothers may be referred to psychiatric providers in the community to provide medication management and pharmacological treatment.

MEETING THE BABY: DELIVERY AND EARLY POSTPARTUM

Civilian mothers can deliver in either a military or a civilian facility depending on their location, wishes, and insurance choice. If the active duty spouse is not deployed or on temporary duty, the male service member has traditionally been granted up to 10 days of paternity leave, depending on the mission of the unit and permission of the commander. On January 29, 2016, paternity leave was increased to 14 days across the DoD (Youssef, 2016).

Once a mother has the baby, the active duty member enrolls his or new infant into DEERS. Most military families typically receive newborn or well childcare through a military pediatrician or primary care provider. Often, the work of parenting is predominately deferred to the dependent spouse to allow the active duty member to focus on their job. Spouses then struggle to adapt to the maternal role, learn how to interact with her infant and adjust to role changes that may include leaving full-time employment to stay home. Other times, a spouse has to adapt to roles of parenting multiple children. In the cases where the active duty member is deployed, the military civilian spouse usually is limited to communicating with her husband (or less commonly her wife) and family via social media.

The Civilian Father/Spouse

There is very limited data on the active duty or civilian male/LGBT spouse. We were not able to find much research specific to struggles of the civilian father and were not able to find any research on perinatal mood or anxiety disorders in male spouses. We did manage to find one article that discussed military and cultural challenges that may affect a male spouse during his transition to fatherhood. Male spouses struggle with going against the cultural image of a masculine warrior that is complimented by the female impact of dependent, supportive spouse. The presence of females as warriors and men as the military spouse challenges the gender dichotomy that is prevalent in the military (Jebo, 2005). Although it has come a long way in gender equality, military culture is traditionally tailored to fit the male active duty service member and female spouse. For instance, culturally, when meeting a military couple for the first time, many individuals in society will assume the male is the active duty member.

In a similar fashion to the transition to fatherhood discussed in Chapter 4, males may prefer to be involved with work where they feel competent versus becoming involved in parenting. For male spouses, the unpredictability of military service leads to the male civilian spouse becoming the primary caregiver, and he will thus require a more flexible career that is lower paying (Jebo, 2005). Male spouses in military families are more likely to work outside the home and feel the societal expectation that they are the "breadwinner" and may feel he is not living up to his expectations as a husband if he is unable to find proper employment (Jebo, 2005). Given the relative "reversal" of gender roles, active duty women married to male civilians may experience guilt related to this role reversal and feel oblicated to be the primary caretaker. As a result, active duty women may engage in behaviors called "maternal gatekeeping" wherein they exert control over the quality and quantity of time their spouse spends with their infant (Pederson & Kilzer, 2013). Maternal gatekeeping theorizes that employed mothers may have a hard time letting go of the traditional mother role and thereby reflexively attempt to maintain control over the couple's division of childcare (Pederson & Kilzer, 2013).

As active duty females may deploy anywhere from 6–12 months postpartum, the male civilian spouse is left to be the main caretaker of his infant during a time critical for infant development wherein he will become the attachment figure. Culturally, the male spouse may be stereotyped when he is out with his infant, as many individuals may hold fast to gender stereotypes and false concepts that only mothers know how to care for babies. Consequently, he may draw lots of attention from others who view him as the "poor dad" struggling to take care of an infant and who question him about where the infant's mother may be. Like fatherhood stereotypes, he may battle the gender stereotype that men do not know how to take care of infants or engage in primary responsibility for children.

The male civilian spouse may face gender role challenges with obtaining support from military programs that are predominately targeted toward female civilian spouses and may have programs only available during the day (Goodman et al., 2013). During deployments, male spouses may not be reached out to by the deploying unit, as it is assumed if he is a man, then he must not be struggling to adapt to his wife's deployment.

The Military Mother

> "I am an active duty Commander, and department head, my husband owns a small business in the States, we decided on a geographical separation overseas to keep the company running since there are not satisfactory jobs overseas. It was now or never to get pregnant. We are very excited because we are pregnant, but we are nervous because I do not have any family or friends here."

Overview

Several decades ago, women were discharged from the military if they became pregnant (Mulhall, 2009; Wahl & Randall, 1996). In contrast, today it is common to see pregnant servicewomen serving throughout the military, including assignments to deployable units (Bucher, 1999). Active duty women have career freedom and opportunities similar to male counterparts; they can deploy at high frequency, work long hard hours, and not think twice about the schedule (Goodman et al., 2013; Taber, 2013). Such a schedule may be suitable for single servicewomen (or married without kids); however, such a mobile career may be difficult for the military mother. As active duty service members, military mothers must manage the demands of active duty service, deal with prolonged separation from family for deployment or training purposes, cope with frequent relocations and long or unpredictable work hours at the same time that they are trying to balance challenges innate to parenthood (Evans & Rosen, 1997; Shumer & Maloney, 2007). As a result, active duty moms often cite feeling as if they have divided loyalties—split between their career and their desire to be good mothers. Given these challenges, many active duty women may struggle with the transition to motherhood and are at risk of developing mood or anxiety disorders during pregnancy or the postpartum period.

Prevalence

The Armed Forces Surveillance Study examined rates of perinatal depression as well as suicidality in active duty women and found 9% of first-time active duty mothers were diagnosed with depression within 12 months of delivery. These women were 42 times more likely to be diagnosed with suicidality (Do et al., 2013). Other, smaller studies that researched the rates of postpartum depression in active duty mothers had broader inclusion criteria and found rates of positive depression screen ranged from 19.5% to 50% among active duty mothers studied (Appolonio & Fingerhut, 2008; O'Boyle, Magann, Ricks, Doyle, & Morrison, 2005).

Considering Motherhood

All branches of military service encourage servicewomen to plan a pregnancy to balance successfully the demands of family responsibilities and military obligations (U.S. Navy, 2007). At any time, a woman can be reassigned to a deployable unit or receive notice that she is to deploy. However, despite the deployment and operational concerns, most active duty pregnancies are not actively prevented, and even with their best intentions, around 54% of pregnancies in active duty women may be unplanned (Grindlay & Grossman, 2013). Pregnancy in military women directly influences their military readiness ad well as impacts readiness of their unit (Grindlay & Grossman, 2013). Because all military services render women non-deployable during their pregnancy, pregnant service members may have physical and job-related duty limitations (Biggs, Douglas, O'Boyle, & Rieg, 2009).

Acceptance of Pregnancy and Commitment to Maternal Role

Once an active duty mother discovers her pregnancy, she is faced with a myriad of changes in her career path. Also, to the psychological acceptance of pregnancy, a pregnant servicewoman has many practical steps she must take upon discovering her pregnancy. In all services, a newly pregnant servicewoman may have a specific time limit from point of diagnosis of pregnancy until she informs her command (U.S. Navy, 2007).

All services require commands to counsel active duty women upon confirmation that she is pregnant and usually address the specific actions a woman must take during pregnancy in preparation for managing dual roles of military and as a mother (U.S. Navy, 2007; USAPHC, 2010). Depending on the service, women are usually given the option to be discharged from the service if they do not desire to continue in military service during pregnancy (U.S. Navy, 2007; USAPHC, 2010). In reality, getting out of the military during pregnancy is not a feasible or desirable option for most servicewomen, as some will have service obligations, while others want to stay in the military or potentially need to stay in as a means of providing for their family.

Once a servicewoman is confirmed pregnant, she is made non-deployable and exempt from body weight and physical fitness standards. Although these limitations are meant to help women, they can also cause psychosocial challenges. For instance, in many services, unit physical training is the norm, and a means to build collegiality and morale. A pregnant service member is exempted from unit physical training, but this exemption may create a real or perceived barrier between herself and rest of her unit. Servicewomen are instructed to perform physical training on their own to account for exercise during pregnancy (US Air Force, 2015). In the Army, there is a new program created to address the social support as well as physical fitness in pregnant service members through the creation of Army Pregnancy/Postpartum Physical Training (PPPT or P3T) program (USAPHC, 2010; Young, 2011). In the P3T program, a mother now can participate in a group to learn holistic fitness, nutrition, and behavioral health principles during pregnancy and postpartum with other pregnant or postpartum active duty soldiers. Unfortunately, given the newness of the program, many smaller/non-deployable bases do not have this option, and pregnant soldiers fall under the old policy of doing their physical training (USAPHC, 2010). The P3T program is discussed more thoroughly in the Appendix on body image/exercise and fitness during/after pregnancy.

Pregnant service members have pregnancy limitations specific to their job as well as limitations on duty hours (Grindlay & Grossman, 2013). Again, these restrictions are meant to protect the military mother and her baby, but this can lead to stigma and consternation from her peers if they feel they have to pull a greater share of the burden—especially since service members frequently feel overtasked/overworked at baseline. As the military is a culture where many individuals develop an identity based on their job in the military, ostracization from their unit will likely contribute to significant emotional upset and distress. Active duty pregnancy restrictions may unintentionally precipitate a hostile work environment for a pregnant servicewoman. If her unit members perceive that she is not pulling her weight, pregnancy limitations may undermine her credibility in the eyes of her male and female peers and generate hostility (Bucher, 1999). In some units, women are fully supported, and their unit rallies around her. In contrast, many other units are still built around the "masculine" image, wherein pregnancy can be seen as a sign of weakness and that a pregnant woman is not fulfilling her duty. In particular, if a servicewoman discovers a pregnancy right before her unit is placed on deployment notice, her peers may assume that she is trying to get out of deployment/work. Women in the military also have to struggle with their internal standard of feeling like they have to work harder and be tougher to be accepted by male colleagues. Women may become frustrated with pregnancy limitations and struggle with guilt related to pregnancy. A pregnant service member who is married to a civilian spouse, may find that her husband's excitement can help compensate for the weak support she may receive from her unit. A service woman may struggle to identify with her maternal role during transition to motherhood if she cannot assimilate the maternal role into servicewoman/warrior role.

A Note about Single Service Member Pregnancies

One particular population to recognize is the single parent—particularly the single servicewoman who becomes unexpectedly pregnant. Although military women may be single parents for a variety of reasons, most often this is outside context of marriage/divorce, and thus single parenthood is fraught with negative stereotypes and judgment. Even though American culture recognizes that many children are born outside the context of marriage, there is still a stereotype and expectation in the military that children are born into a marital unit, unless there is divorce. Single women may be viewed as a "burden" on the unit, where others feel they have to make up for what they are unable to do. Commands are encouraged to give single parents extra support, given the understanding that they may not have the social support in the family or from the unit. In other cases, active duty servicewomen are married to active duty men, but due to needs of military, they are separated from their spouse. These women are geographically "single" and may have to endure pregnancy by themselves and require the same support and understanding as that of a single mother.

MENTAL HEALTH CHALLENGES IN PREGNANCY

Military woman are at an elevated risk of depression in pregnancy and postpartum. Factors that increase the risk for depression include social isolation, coping with undesired pregnancy, unresolved psychological trauma from childhood, relationship challenges with a marital partner (or father of the infant), as well as struggling with work demands. When active duty women become depressed, they may discount this as fatigue due to pregnancy and ignore warning signs. They may be worried about how their peers perceive them. Some servicewomen do not want to be pregnant, and in some cases may deny the pregnancy. There have been instances where a servicewoman found the "abortion pill" on the internet and tried to stop her pregnancy. As DoD does not pay for elective abortions, a pregnant soldier who does not want to be pregnant has two choices: seek treatment in the community on her finances, or continue the pregnancy (Grindlay & Grossman, 2013).

In the Army, a servicewoman cannot be stationed overseas during pregnancy, and this can lead to a last-minute reassignment. At this time, there are no identifiers for a pregnant servicewoman that can prevent her from being stationed at a highly deployable unit. This means that a servicewoman can be pulled from an overseas assignment just to be sent to a military unit that has incredibly high operation tempo with deployment already pending. Women who are already suffering depression during pregnancy, especially if it causes performance deficits, have a very high risk of relapse in postpartum. Sending them to another unit means taking a servicewoman away from whatever source of support she has, whatever behavioral health and obstetric therapeutic alliance has been established and she has to start all over. Depending on the service, soon after birth, a servicewoman is expected to deploy in the Army, this can be as little as 6 months, while the remainder of services has given a 12-month deferment. During pregnancy, depressed servicewomen can be placed on a temporary profile at the discretion of a behavioral health provider. The behavioral health provider can put a temporary profile requesting deferment/cancelation of PCS order for stabilization. In the Army, there are general policies that *no* service member can change duty stations if they are unstable in behavioral health treatment. Chapter 13 goes into more details of true experiences of active duty mothers who struggled with depression during pregnancy.

MEETING THE BABY AND BECOMING A MOTHER

Active duty women usually give birth within the military treatment facility unless obstetric treatment is not available and they are referred to a network provider. Maternity leave previously varied dependent on the services. Over the past years, maternity leave was traditionally 6 weeks. In 2015, the U.S. Air Force doubled maternity leave to 12 weeks, and the Navy tripled maternity leave to 18 weeks. (Air Force Public Affairs, 2015; Losey, 2015; Sahadi, 2015) Leaving the Army as the only remaining service to have only 6 weeks. Fortunately, in January 2016, the Pentagon decided to make all maternity leave even across the board, requiring the Navy/Marines to scale back leave from 18 to 12 weeks, which would allow the Army to increase to 12 weeks (Chalfant, 2016; Youssef, 2016).

After maternity leave, a mother is expected to return to full duty and meet physical fitness standards within 6–12 months depending on the service (Air Force Public Affairs, 2015). Time off after delivery is designed to allow an active duty mother time to bond with her infant and start to learn tasks of mothering. Once she returns to work, she has to get to balance various social roles, but only maternity leave is protected time wherein she can learn to become a mother. During this time, active duty moms may breastfeed and make a decision if they desire to breastfeed/pump once they return to work (Roche-Paull, 2015). Recently, TRICARE has helped encourage breastfeeding for active duty moms as well as dependent moms by covering the cost of breast pumps, which can help a mother be more inclined to continue breastfeeding and pumping at work. Some mothers have actually brought breast pumps on deployment and shipped breastmilk home (Buchatz, 2015). At this time, some women struggle with accepting that they have to go back to work. If they were proficient at their job, struggling with tasks of motherhood may lead to them feeling incompetent. As the active duty member, they may feel like they should not ask for help.

MENTAL HEALTH CHALLENGES IN THE EARLY POSTPARTUM PERIOD

Like civilian mothers, active duty mothers may fear seeking treatment, believing it will negatively affect their career, or they fear they will be seen as weak by unit members. Similar to civilian spouses, an active duty mother will most likely have her newborn's care at the military treatment facility. If her unit was not supportive during pregnancy, she might feel weak for not being proficient at motherhood. If her unit was supportive, she might feel like she has to be "supermom" and be an outstanding service member as well as the outstanding mother. Unfortunately, there is only so much energy she can devote to both roles, and she may end up feeling exhausted. In a similar fashion to Masked Male Depression, the active duty mother may worry about showing any emotions and struggle with alexithymia. If she did not have positive female role models, she may feel guilty asking for help and feel guilty about not being able to mother instinctively. Once she returns to work, she may feel like she has to make up for "lost time" and may take on too much, not allowing herself time to adjust to changes in her role at work, to recognize her dual role as well as adapt to motherhood.

Active duty mothers have to adapt to the physical and mental challenge of returning to a pre-pregnancy fitness level. Although losing baby weight is a common goal for all postpartum mothers, for active duty women, their career depends on it. This common stressor regarding return to pre-baby fitness levels as well as returning to weight standards can lead to siginificant distress. A more extreme example that illustrated how this fear of not "returning to normal" can affect a woman's mental health in active duty moms was highlighted in 2013 when an active duty Air Force staff sergeant was in danger of not passing her postpartum physical fitness test and feared she would be kicked out of the Air Force. Struggling with this fear, as well as coping with the challenges of being a new mother (and probably postpartum depression), this staff sergeant recruited an individual to stab her in the stomach so she would not have to take her fitness test (Pawlyk, 2013). While cases like above are very rare, it does illuminate the importance of recognizing concerns about body image.

Years Following Childbirth

All services expect active duty mothers to balance the role of parenthood with their military career. Active duty mothers are required by each service to make arrangements for childcare to cover regular working hours, duty, exercises and pre-deployment operations (US Navy, 2007). All single service members and dual-military couples with eligible family members are responsible for initiating a formalized family care plan per reference (US Air Force, 2015; USAPHC, 2010; US Navy, 2007). A completed family care plan will certify that family members will be cared for during the service member's absence. It will also identify the designated legal guardian of the eligible family member(s), as well as logistical, relocation, and financial arrangements.

Given the challenges balancing work/home life, active duty mothers can struggle with adjusting to new interpersonal roles and developing a motherhood identity. A military mother may feel like she has to sacrifice her career for motherhood and consequently become bitter at her infant or bitter at the military. Once back at work, she must have childcare arranged, including backup childcare. Depending on which service, she will enter into the pre-deployment phase and has to be prepared for deployment on a moment's notice. Deployment means separation from her child. Particularly, if deploying soon after birth, this means the mother has to miss one of the most critical periods in her infant's life, leading to disrupted attachment. Even if she has a supportive spouse/family, she may feel guilty for being away from her child, especially because society often expects women to be the main caretakers of children. These challenges have led to some women getting out of military and choosing to stay home (Evans & Rosen, 1997). In the case of dual military spouse—this can then lead to guilt/

sense of dissatisfaction that they had to give up a career for their child. Other times, a woman may become resentful of her family if pregnancy/postpartum led to missed opportunities to deploy/advance her career (Appolonio & Fingerhut, 2008; Rychnovsky, 2006). To address these issues, the military services began with a pilot program in 2012 called the Career Interruption Program. This allows active duty men or women to take up to a 2-year deferment with expected payback to follow career aspirations or start a family.

The Military Father

> "I am not sure whom to address this to since I am a Marine stationed on an Army base. My wife gave birth 2.5 months ago, and we moved not long after that (a move just before the birth as well). She has become very depressed since arriving here. I am wondering where I can find her some help, as she is starting to feel hopeless, and I am getting very worried about her."

In Chapter 4, we discussed fatherhood and psychological aspects/challenges associated with fatherhood. Given the recognition of the importance of fatherhood, there has been increasing recognition of the plight of military dads. Military fathers have traditionally been stereotyped as dads who work, while the dependent mother was responsible for care of military children with fathers intermittently involved. Military fathers may be married to civilian spouses, married to active duty women or functioning as single dads. In dual-active-duty families, military fathers are commonly culturally expected to defer primary childcare to their wife, despite both parents being military. Military fathers who try to take a more active role may feel like they do not get equal support.

The responsibilities of military service can complicate the development of father–child attachment (Lee et al., 2013). Extended deployments that occur during infancy and childhood can disrupt a father's ability to bond to his children (Lee et al., 2013). Additionally, when not deployed, fathers may be separated from children due to "geo-baching" discussed in the previous chapter, or due to duty-related training responsibilities (Lee et al., 2013). Studies of first-time fathers have reported that men desire more information across pregnancy and early parenthood, especially regarding potential changes in their relationship with their romantic partner (Lee et al., 2013). In research studies, fathers have been found to rely on informal sources of information such as friends and co-workers. Military fathers did not admit to seeking much help in a community—in one part because most support for postpartum is geared toward mothers, and they had a high chance of being the only male in an all-female environment (Lee et al., 2013).

Commitment to Fatherhood

Given the statistic that over 49% of pregnancies are unplanned, many military fathers may feel unprepared as they enter fatherhood. An expectant father may thus revisit his childhood and his relationship with his father. During this time, an expectant father may realize he needs to look beyond his family to understand what makes a "good father" (Barnes & Balber, 2007). Many military fathers are motivated to be excellent fathers and desire to provide a better life for their child (Walsh et al., 2014). The standard antepartum parenting classes may not be sufficient for fathers, especially as research has found that antenatal education is not as helpful to dads as it is for expectant moms (May & Fletcher, 2013). In studies on antenatal education, mothers and fathers were more likely to have better postnatal health when they attend antenatal care that is delivered to couples and models of shared infant care, addresses couple relationships and sensitizes men to experiences of their wives (May & Fletcher, 2013).

In military fathers, key challenges in preparation for fatherhood include defining the co-parenting relationship, developing identity as father and defining the co-parenting role (Dayton, Walsh, Muzik, Erwin, & Rosenblum, 2014). In studies, military fathers found information on how to co-parent and strategies to support their partner were most helpful, as well as information on a woman's physical and emotional changes during pregnancy (Lee et al., 2013). Fathers also desired to connect and learn from other fathers, especially fathers who had experienced deploying and reuniting with their family (Walsh et al., 2014).

Meeting the Baby

Over the past three decades, men have become a regular presence in delivery rooms and involved during the pregnancy and birth of their children (Schachman, 2010). Paternal involvement during childbirth may serve to facilitate the childbirth process, enhance both maternal and paternal self-esteem, strengthen the couple relationship and facilitate the parent–infant attachment (May & Fletcher, 2013).

Today, over 90% of fathers attend the birth of their children (Schachman, 2010). For many men, the transition to fatherhood must include being involved with birth (Schachman, 2010). In a sociocultural analysis of fatherhood, the research found that the sense of responsibility and protectiveness innate to fatherhood emerge immediately after birth (Schachman, 2010). Being present at birth allows men a chance to feel connected to their newborn and start the father–infant bond (Schachman, 2010). Military fathers who are stateside can usually attend the birth of their children and are also granted up to 10 days of paternity leave. The paternity policy was recently changed in January 2016 when the Pentagon made maternity leave 12 weeks uniform across the services, accompanied by increasing paternity leave to 14 weeks (Chalfant, 2016; McAvoy, 2015).

As discussed in Chapter 4, fathers have previously been absent for the birth of their children, and only after the last decade have fathers "reappeared" to become present at birth. Unfortunately, in the military, many fathers are absent from the birth of their children due to military obligations (Schachman, 2010).

There have been several research studies discussing perception and experience of fatherhood while deployed (MacDermid, Schwarz, Faber, Adkins, & Mishkind, 2004; Schachman, 2013; Walsh et al., 2014). Many of these studies were constructed on the premise that military fathers felt an obligation to protect their wives and children, and hence their absence from birth and family interfered with their ability to fulfill this role (Schachman, 2010; Walsh et al., 2014). Leading up to delivery, deployed fathers often were worried and consumed about the safety of their baby and their wife. In particular, deployed fathers often imagined their presence at birth as a way to restore order to a dangerous situation. Being absent from delivery contributed to deployed fathers fretting about their wives not having enough support at delivery (Schachman, 2010). Deployed fathers also felt guilty about what they perceived as a "lost opportunity" to participate in a special moment of a critical life transition (Schachman, 2010; Walsh et al., 2014) and subsequently felt guilty about feeling like they "chose" their career over their family (Schachman, 2010; Walsh, et al., 2014). Military fathers struggled with their military career and family challenges and expressed concern that if they got out of the military, then they would be without a job or insurance for their pregnant wife, which, in turn, would lead to an even greater predicament (Schachman, 2010).

Even if fathers are present at the birth of their children, they may experience difficulties connecting to their babies when they are not the primary caregivers or providing most of the active parenting, especially in infancy (Lee et al., 2013). For example, some fathers felt disconnected because the mother was breastfeeding and primary source of food/comfort, making them have difficulty finding a way to connect to the baby (Lee et al., 2013).

Transitioning to New Roles

One important aspect of transitioning to new roles includes an opportunity for a time at home with the infant and spouse. For non-deployed fathers, this opportunity is present during paternity leave. New fathers may feel exhausted and must learn to adapt to the challenges of parenting and fatherhood, as well as adjust to the role of a military father (Willerton, Schwarz, Wadsorth, & Oglesby, 2011). Part of this adjustment includes understanding different stages of an infant's development (Lee et al., 2013). For instance, fathers may struggle to know how to soothe a fussy infant and not understand that infants tend to have a fussy period each day (Lee et al., 2013). In this instance, experienced military fathers suggested they would find it helpful to be reassured that persistent difficulty in comforting their infant or establishing a sleep schedule did not mean they were doing something wrong (Lee et al., 2013). Military fathers had to learn how to adjust their expectations from military life to family life (Walsh et al., 2014) and learn how to adjust to the unpredictability of a child's behavior. Military fathers also want to get to express emotions and provide nurturing care to their children and may defer affection and nurturing to their partner due to difficulties expressing emotion (Walsh et al., 2014). Another common skill father's desire is to learn to control their temper during high-stress moments (Walsh et al., 2014).

Mental Health Challenges for Military Fathers

As discussed in Chapter 4, new fathers are at risk for perinatal mood and anxiety disorders and can develop paternal postpartum depression. Due to military culture that prides suppression of emotions, military fathers are more likely to struggle with alexithymia, expression of emotions and seeking treatment. Fathers who are returning from deployment may feel guilty for missed time and feel like an "imposter in my home." A military father struggles to balance demands of the military with the needs of his family. If his wife is struggling with depression, the needs of the military may prevent him from fully trying to share the burden/assist his spouse in recovery. He may be afraid to approach command for fear of being perceived as weak. Military fathers hesitate to seek help from commands, fearing that commanders will not understand. Despite this concern, many who do seek command support may discover that command is very supportive. Similar to employment in the civilian environment, the support commanders/leaders render will differ depending on each individual. Military leaders who are also fathers tend to be more supportive/understanding, while others may have little understanding/compassion for new fathers.

The Military Marriage

In addition to risks to the mother, postpartum depression often leads to difficulties with interpersonal relationships, including social relationships, marital relationships, mother–child relationships, as well as negative consequences overall to the family unit.

Research has also shown that maternal depression affects a woman's perception of the quality of her intimate relationships and social supports. In particular, postpartum depression has been associated with increased rates of marital conflict, separation, and divorce which can then exacerbate maternal depression. When a military spouse faces parenting alone, she may develop a distorted view of marriage. There have been cases when military spouses were on the verge of divorcing their spouse because they did not perceive any help. Male spouses of active duty moms may become resentful that they are doing more of the work than a military spouse. They also may resent long hours/deployments that spouse has, especially if their childhood mother stayed home.

Mental health problems (especially perinatal mental health) in active duty spouses lead to a decrease in service member's support during deployment/reintegration into family and civilian life (Verdeli et al., 2011). Military service members (spouses of women with postpartum depression) have reported increased stress, and less marital satisfaction, which can lead to/contribute to mental health disorder in the service member. Overall, research has found that service members with dissatisfied spouses are more likely to leave the military, thus contributing to decreased readiness as well as a reduction in retention of a robust and experienced military force (Verdeli et al., 2011). In addition to impact on retention and readiness, perinatal depression in either spouse may lead to higher risk of domestic violence and child maltreatment. Increased risk of domestic abuse/violence occurs when one parent struggles with mental illness, especially if the parent who is struggling is the main caretaker of the children. In additional to marital relationships being affected, perinatal mental health challenges also affect parenting abilities and mental health of infants/children (Paley, Lester, & Mogil, 2013).

The Military Infant/Child

The mental health of children exists in the context of family relationships. Infants and children of military families have unique considerations during the perinatal period (Lieberman & Van Horn, 2013). In the military family, attachment and bonding in infancy are challenged by the frequent geographical separation for assignments, training and deployments (Boris & Zeanah 1999).

Prenatal

In Chapter 3, we discussed how maternal stress impacts infant growth and development in utero. Active duty mothers are exposed to additional stress during pregnancy given the nature of their job. Dependent spouses are also exposed to stress, especially if their military husband is deployed during pregnancy or childbirth. Mothers who are stressed/depressed during pregnancy can have decreased bonding, decreased attachment or poor acceptance of pregnancy and difficulty committing to the parenting role. For military fathers, if they are deployed during pregnancy, they miss out on opportunities to transition to the fatherhood role and begin to imagine themselves as a father.

Postpartum

Mothers who are anxious or depressed in the postpartum period have increased difficulty bonding to their infant. Both active duty mothers and fathers may be reluctant to seek assistance, due to fear of stigma. Parent mental health challenges will usually lead to problems with parent–infant relationship. Add to this the stressors of a military move and frequent absences, and infant and young children may have difficulty developing a sense of trust. The absent parent (gone for military training/deployment), as well as the parent who remains taking care of the homefront, may have challenges investing emotional time and energy into developing a parent–infant relationship. The at home parent may feel overwhelmed and struggle with basic caretaking aspects of parenting and running a household. The absent parent is removed from infant's life during a critical time in development. The military parent may miss birthdays, milestones and special moments that create lasting memories. The at-home parent may be taxed with his or her issues and not be able to emotionally attune to their child, leading a child to be unable to engage effectively with either parent.

If parent–child attachment bonds are disrupted over a long period, children can have a hard time viewing their caregiver as a source of safety and security (Chandra et al., 2010). A child whose parent is frequently deployed within the first 5 years of its life leads to repeated losses of an attachment figure, which can subsequently lead to difficulties attaching to that parent (Chandra et al., 2010). The child may feel rejected by the deployed member and not able to connect with the distressed caregiver at home. Once service members return home, children can be very sensitive to a parent leaving again and can become anxious about a parent even dressing in uniform (McFarlane, 2009).

Summary

In this chapter, we have discussed how military culture and the military health system can affect the experience of pregnancy and parenting among various roles in the military family system. In the next section, we will discuss both non-pharmacological treatments followed by pharmacological treatments followed by discussing specific intervention models in the various specialty fields in military medicine.

References

Air Force Public Affairs. (2015). PT Exemptions, Dwell Time for New AF Mothers Increase to One Year. Air Force Print New TODAY. Retrieved from http://www.afpc.af.mil/news/story_print.asp?id=123453477

Allen, A., Flinn, A., & Moore, W. (2007). The 81st medical group obstetrics and gynecology flight's role during hurricane Katrina. *Military Medicine, 172*(2), 199–201. Retrieved from https://www.ncbi.nlm.nih.gov/pubmed/?term=Allen%2C+A.%2C+Flinn%2C+A.%2C+%26+Moore%2C+W.+(2007).+The+81st+medical+group+obstetrics+and+gynecology+flight%E2%80%99s+role+during+hurricane+Katrina.

Appolonio, K. K., & Fingerhut, R. (2008). Postpartum depression in a military sample. *Military Medicine, 173*(11), 1085–1091.

Barnes, D., & Balber, L. (2007). *The Journey to Parenthood: Myths, Realities and What Really Matters*. Oxon, UK: Radcliffe Publishing.

Biggs, R., Douglas, B., O'Boyle, A., & Rieg, T. (2009). The impact of pregnancy on the individual and military organization: A postpartum active duty survey. *Military Medicine, 174*(1), 61–75.

Blue Star Families. (2014). *Military Family Lifestyle Survey: Comprehensive Report.* Falls Church, VA: Department of Research and Policy. Retrieved from http://vets.syr.edu/wp-content/uploads/2014/01/BSFReportComprehensiveReport.pdf

Boris, N., & Zeanah, C. (1999). Disturbances and disorders of attachment in infancy: An overview. *Infant Mental Health Journal, 20*(1), 1–9.

Buchatz, A. (2015). New Tricare Policy Gives Free Breast Pumps. *Military.com.* Retrieved from http://www.military.com/daily-news/2015/06/05/new-tricare-policy-gives-free-breast-pumps.html (Accessed on 28 January 2016).

Bucher, M. (1999). *The Impact of Pregnancy on Army Readiness.* AU/ACSC/016/1994–04, Alabama: Maxwell Air Force Base.

Chalfant, M. (2016). Pentagon gives military moms 12 weeks maternity leave: Walks back SecNav policy change from last year. *The Washington Free Beacon.* Retrieved from http://freebeacon.com/national-security/pentagon-gives-military-moms-12-weeks-maternity-leave/ (Accessed on 28 January 2016).

Chandra, A., Lara-Cinisomo, S., Jaycox, L., Tanielian, T., Burns, R., Ruder, T., & Han, B. (2010). Children on the homefront: The experience of children from military families. *Pediatrics, 125*, 16–25. doi:10.1542/peds.2009–1180

Danielson, R. (2010). Childbirth, Deployment and Diagnoses of Mental Disorders among Active Component Women. Retrieved from Armed Forces Health Surveillance Center: www.afhsc.mil/documents/pubs/msmrs/2010/v17_n11.pdf

Dayton, C., Walsh, T., Muzik, M., Erwin, M., & Rosenblum, K. (2014). Strong, safe, and secure: Negotiating early fathering and military service across the deployment cycle. *Infant Mental Health Journal, 35*(5), 509–520.

Do, T., Hu, Z., Otto, J., & Rohrbeck, P. (2013). Depression and suicidality during the postpartum period after first time deliveries, active component service women and dependent spouses, U.S. Armed Forces, 2007–2012. *Medical Surveillance Monthly Reports (MSMR).* Retrieved from http://www.health.mil/Military-Health-Topics/Health-Readiness/Armed-Forces-Health-Surveillance-Branch/Reports-and-Publications/~/link.aspx?_id=534E26BD8E5D4ECC8CAA8ABA47679691&_z=z

Evans, M. A., & Rosen, L. (1997). Pregnancy planning and the impact on work climate, psychological well-being, and work effort in the military. *Journal of Occupational Health Psychology, 2*(4), 353–361.

Goodman, P., Turner, A., Agazio, J., Throop, M., Padden, D., Greiner, S., & Hillier, S. (2013). Deployment of military mothers: Supportive and nonsupportive military programs, processes and policies. *Military Medicine, 178*(7), 729–734. Retrieved from https://www.ncbi.nlm.nih.gov/pubmed/23820345

Grindlay, K., & Grossman, D. (2013). Unintended pregnancy among active-duty women in the United States military, 2008. *Obstetrics and Gynecology, 121*(2), 241–246. Retrieved from http://10.1097/AOG.0b013e31827c616e

Jebo, Jennifer. (2005). An Untraditional Life: Male Spouses of Female Military Personnel. Dissertation submitted to Virginia Polytechnic Institute and State University, 29 April. Blacksburg, VA.

Haas, D. M., Pazdernik, L. A., & Olsen, C. H. (2005). A cross-sectional survey of the relationship between partner deployment and stress in pregnancy during wartime. *Women's Health Issues, 15*, 48–54.

Lee, S., Neugut, T., Rosenblum, Tolman, R., Travis, W., & Walker, M. (2013). Sources of parenting support in early fatherhood: Perspective of United States Air Force Members. *Children and Youth Services Review, 35*, 908–915.

Levine, J., Bukowinski, A., Sevick, C., Mehlhaff, K., & Conlin, A. (2015). Postpartum depression and timing of spousal military deployment relative to pregnancy and delivery. *Archives Gynecology & Obstetrics,* 292(3), 549–558. doi: 10.1007/s00404-015-3672-7.

Lieberman, A., & Van Horn, P. (2013). *Psychotherapy with Infants and Young Children: Repairing the Effects of Stress and Trauma on Early Attachment.* New York: The Guildford Press.

Losey, S. (2015). Air Force gives new mom three years off. *Air Force Times.* Retrieved from http://www.airforcetimes.com/story/military/careers/air-force/2015/03/08/air-force-new-mom-three-years-off/24505427/

MacDermid, S., Schwarz, R., Faber, A., Adkins, J., & Mishkind, M. (2004). Fathers on the front lines. In W. Marsiglio, K. Roy, & G. L. Fox (Eds.), *Situated Fathering: A Focus on Physical and Social Spaces.* Boulder, CO: Rowman & Littlefield. Retrieved from https://www.mfri.purdue.edu/. . ./FathersOnTheFrontLines.pdf

May, C., & Fletcher, R. (2013). Preparing fathers for the transition to parenthood: Recommendations for the content of antenatal education. *Midwifery, 29*, 474–478.

McAvoy, A. (2015). CNO: Service considering expanding paternity leave. *Navy Times.* Retrieved from http://www.navytimes.com/story/military/2015/10/14/navy-chief-service-considering-expanding-paternity-leave/73914060

McFarlane, A. (2009). Military deployment: The impact on children and family adjustment and need for care. *Current Opinion in Psychiatry,* 22, 369–373.

Mulhall, E. (2009). Women Warriors: Supporting She "Who Has Borne the Battle". NYS Health Foundation. Retrieved from http://nyshealthfoundation.org/resources-and-reports/resource/women-warriors-supporting-she-who-has-borne-the-battle

O'Boyle, A., Magann, E., Ricks, R., Doyle., M., & Morrison, J. (2005). Depression screening in the pregnant soldier wellness program. *Southern Medical Journal, 98*(4), 416–418. Retrieved from https://www.ncbi.nlm.nih.gov/pubmed/?term=Depression+screening+in+the+pregnant+soldier+wellness+program

Paley, B., Lester, P., & Mogil, C. (2013). Family systems and ecological perspective on the impact of deployment on military families. *Clinical Child and Family Psychology Review, 16*(3), 245–265. Springer. Published online, 13 June 2013. doi: 10.1007/s10567-013-0138-y. Retrieved from https://www.ncbi.nlm.nih.gov/pubmed/?term=Paley%2C+B.%2C+Lester%2C+P.%2C+%26+Mogil%2C+C.+(2013).+Family+systems+and+ecologicial+perspective+on+the+impact+of+deployment+on+military+families

Pawlyk, O. (2013). Former staff sergeant stabbed to avoid PT test. *Air Force Times.* Retrieved from http://archive.airforcetimes.com/article/20130722/NEWS06/307220031/Former-staff-sergeant-stabbed-avoid-PT-test

Pederson, D., & Kilzer, G. (2013). Work-to-family conflict and the maternal gatekeeping of dual-earner mothers with young children. *Journal of Family Economic Issues.* Springer. Published online, 30 August 2013. Retrieved from http://link.springer.com/article/10.1007/s10834-013-9370-3

Robrecht, D., Millegan, J., Leventis, L., Crescitelli, J.-B., & McLay, R. (2008). Spousal military deployment as risk factor for postpartum depression. *The Journal of Reproductive Medicine, 53*(11), 860–864. Retrieved from https://www.ncbi.nlm.nih.gov/pubmed/19097519

Roche-Paull, R. (2015). Breastfeeding in Combat Boots. http://breastfeedingincombatboots.com

Rychnovsky, J. (2006). Screening for postpartum depression in military women with the postpartum depression screening scale. *Military Medicine, 171*(11), 1100–1104. Retrieved from https://www.ncbi.nlm.nih.gov/pubmed/17153549

Sahadi, J. (2015). U.S. navy triples paid maternity leave to 18 weeks. *CNN Money*. July 2, 2015. New York. Retrieved from http://money.cnn.com/2015/07/02/pf/navy-paid-maternity-leave/index.html

Schachman, K. (2010). Online fathering: The experience of first-time fatherhood in combat deployed troops. *Nursing Research, 59*(1), 11–17.

Schachman, K., & Lindsey, L. (2013). A resilience perspective of postpartum depressive symptomatology in military wives. *Journal of Obstetric and Gynecological Nursing, 42*, 157–167. doi:10.1111/1552–6909.12007

Shumer, C., & Maloney, C. (2007). *Helping Military Moms Balance Family and Longer Deployments*. United States Senate: Joint Economics Committee. Retrieved from http://www.jec.senate.gov/archive/Documents/Reports/MilitaryMoms05.11.07Final.pdf

Smith, D. C., Munroe, M. L., Foglia, L. M., Nielsen, P. E., & Deering, S. H. (2010). Effects of deployment on depression screening scores in pregnancy at an army military treatment facility. *Obstetrics and Gynecology, 116*(3), 679–683.

Spieker, A. (2012). *Spousal Military Deployment during Pregnancy and Adverse Birth Outcomes*. (Master's Thesis in Publish Health), University of Washington, Seattle. Retrieved from https://digital.lib.washington.edu/researchworks/bitstream/handle/1773/20534/Spieker_washington_0250O_10207.pdf?sequence=1&isAllowed=y

Spooner, S., Rastle, M., & Elmore, K. (2012). Maternal depression screening during prenatal and postpartum care at a navy and marine corps military treatment facility. *Military Medicine, 177*(10), 1208–1211. Retrieved from https://www.ncbi.nlm.nih.gov/pubmed/23113449

Taber, N. (2013). A composite life history of a mother in the military: Storying gendered experiences. *Women's Studies International Forum, 37*, 16–25.

Tarney, C., Berry-Caban, C., Jain, R., Kelly, M., Sewell, M., & Wilson, K. (2015). Association of spousal deployment on pregnancy outcomes in a U.S. population study. *Obstetrics and Gynecology, 126*(3), 569–574.

Thomas, N., Sleath, B. L. Jackson, E. West, S. & Gaynes, B. (2008). Survey of characteristics and treatment preferences for physicians treating postpartum depression in the general medical setting. Community Mental Health Journal. 44(1).: 47-56. Epub 2007 Oct 24. PMID:17957469 doi:10.1007/s10597-007-9108-5

US Air Force. (2015). Air Force Instruction 44–102: Medical Care Management. Retrieved from www.e-publishing.af.mil

US Army Public Health Command (USPHC). (2010). *A Guide to Female Solider Readiness*. Aberdeen Proving Ground, MD: USACHPPM. Retrieved from https://www.pdhealth.mil/dcs/downloads/GFSR.pdf

US NAVY. (2007). *OPNAV Instruction 6000.1C: Navy Guidelines Concerning Pregnancy and Parenthood*. 2000 Navy Pentagon, Washington, DC: Office of the Chief of Naval Operations.

Verdeli, H., Baily, C., Vousoura, E., Belser, A., Manos, G., & Singla, D. (2011). The case for treating depression in military spouses. *Journal of Family Psychology, 25*(4), 488–496. doi:10.1037/a0024525

Wahl, C., & Randall, V. (1996). Military women as wives and mothers. *Women's Health Issues, 6*(6), 315–319.

Walsh, T., Dayton, C., Erwin, M., Muzik, M., Busuito, A., & Rosenblum, K. (February 2014). Fathering after military deployment: Parenting challenges and goals of fathers of young children. *Health & Social Work, 39*(1), 35–44. Retrieved from https://www.ncbi.nlm.nih.gov/pubmed/24693602.

Willerton, E., Schwarz, R., Wadsorth, M., & Oglesby, M. (2011). Military fathers' perspectives on involvement. *Journal of Family Psychology, 25*(4), 521–530.

Young, Lisa. (2011). Army Pregnancy/Postpartum Physical Training Program Overview Brief. United States Army Public Health Command (USAPHC). Retrieved from http://phc.amedd.army.mil/topics/healthyliving/al/Pages/ArmyPregnancyPostpartumPhysicalTrainingProgram.aspx.

Youssef, N. (2016). Pentagon's progressive revolution adds more maternity leave: Servicewomen will now get 12 weeks of paid under another new social change by Secretary Ash Carter. Many officers, steeped in tradition, worries he's moving too fast though. *The Daily Beast.* Retrieved from http://www.thedailybeast.com/articles/2016/01/28/pentagon-s-progressive-revolution-adds-more-maternity-leave.html (Accessed on 28 January, 2016).

Part III

From Diagnosis to Treatment

Chapter 7

Non-pharmacological Treatment Modalities

Valerie Jobrack and Melinda A. Thiam

Much of this book has discussed the challenges and consequences of perinatal mood and anxiety disorders both in the general population as well as the military population. Effective, evidence-based treatments exist, and these include both pharmacological and non-pharmacological treatments (COPE Guidelines, 2011; Goodman, 2009; NICE Guidelines, 2014; Yonkers et al., 2012). Obstetricians, pediatricians and family medicine providers can help screen and potentially diagnose perinatal mood and anxiety disorders, but they must refer to specialty care for most of these treatments. This chapter will address non-pharmacological treatments, and the next subsequent chapter will discuss pharmacological and somatic therapies. Treatment recommendations for both pharmacological and non-pharmacological treatment depend on the following factors: nature of the mental health disorder; the severity of symptoms; a woman's previous response to treatment; and the support, resources and desires of the woman (Williams, 2014). For women with mild to moderate symptoms of depression/anxiety disorders, non-pharmacological treatments are recommended before pharmacological treatment (Williams, 2014).

Barriers to Care

There are many treatment barriers to women with perinatal mental health disorders who attempt to seek help (Williams, 2014). Common barriers include themes of limited availability, social acceptability and accessibility (Verdeli et al., 2011; Williams, 2014). Specific examples of variables that prevent mothers from disclosing symptoms are shown in Table 7.1.

Availability

Availability of care addresses financial and logistical barriers such as time constraints, transportation or childcare (Goodman, 2009). In the military population, military service members and their spouses have access to TRICARE, so they have insurance coverage. However, there is limited availability of behavioral health providers nationwide, let alone providers with expertise

Table 7.1 Variables that Prevent Disclosure of Perinatal Mood Disorder Symptoms (Kleiman, 2009; Williams, 2014)

- Minimization of symptoms and belief symptoms will go away (denial)
- Mother's inability to mobilize self
- Desire for quick fix
- Cost
- Lack of childcare and transportation to get to appointment (geographical isolation)
- Failure to differentiate between symptoms consistent with normal adjustment versus symptoms signifying need for mental health symptoms
- Stigma (guilt, shame, and judgement—associated with mental illness)
- Not knowing that obstetrician/another doctor can help
- Afraid of being "labeled" as depressed
- "Fear of baby being taken away"
- Concerns about confidentiality

*Adapted from text in Kleiman, K. (2009), *Therapy and the Postpartum Woman: Notes on Healing Postpartum Depression for Clinicians and the Women Who Seek Their Help*. New York: Routledge, and Williams, J. (2014), *Best Practice Guidelines for Mental Health Disorders in the Perinatal Period. BC Reproductive Mental Health Program & Perinatal Services BC*. Vancouver BC: Perinatal Services BC.

in perinatal mental health. Although a few large military medical centers have integrated treatment, most military treatment centers do not. Due to the shortage of mental health professionals in military medical centers, dependent children and spouses are typically referred off the post. Off post treatment may require a long wait time (in particular for medication) and TRICARE is not universally accepted insurance. Furthermore, while both the Department of Defense and Veterans Affairs have programs to monitor quality of care, there is usually minimal oversight to monitor quality of care provided by network providers. Therapists such as clinical social workers, psychologists, and licensed professional counselors may be available, but many of these providers are not well versed in some of the unique aspects of military perinatal mental health. One study of the Army population found that of the mental health providers listed on TRICARE website, only 25% of these providers were accepting new patients (Collins & MacDermid-Wadsworth, 2014). This number decreased if there were a high number of deployed soldiers in the area (Collins & MacDermid-Wadsworth, 2014).

Accessibility

Although military families have limited availability of care, even care that is available may not be accessible. Military family members and active duty parents may have logistical barriers such as lack of time, lack of transportation, and lack of childcare. Military life often requires frequent geographic moves; frequent relocation leads to disruption of support networks and often location away from extended family. After relocation, service members and their families must re-establish treatment with new health care providers and find new community resources in their new community (Johnson, Knauss, Faran, & Ban, 2014).

Social Acceptability/Attitudinal Barriers

Mothers frequently fear seeking treatment for mental health challenges and often fear that they would be considered a "bad" mother if they ever admitted their depressed thoughts to others (Kleiman, 2009). When military spouses struggle with or experience depression in the postpartum period, they may simultaneously feel overwhelmed about new motherhood and have internal role expectations that they should "handle everything" related to their own health and parenting, especially if their spouse is deployed during this postpartum period (Verdeli et al., 2011). Mothers with perinatal mood or anxiety disorders may struggle with a sense of shame and inadequacy as they compare themselves to other new mothers they see in civilian and military community who appear like they "have it all together" (Kleiman, 2009). Both military and civilian mothers struggle with internal stigma against mental illness and may also fear how they would be perceived by their primary care provider (COPE guidelines, 2011).

Treatment Overview

There are many approaches to treatment for perinatal mood and anxiety disorders. See Table 7.2 or a list of generalized treatment approaches in pregnancy and evidence-based therapies that have the increasing intensity of treatment, starting with basics and moving towards inpatient hospitalization. The standard approach would be to match treatment intensity to the severity of mood or anxiety symptoms. Basic treatments include psychoeducation and self-care, followed by psychotherapies, then consideration for pharmacological treatment (COPE Guidelines, 2011; Williams, 2014). See Table 7.2.

Psychoeducation

The goal of psychoeducation is to help women and their families understand their symptoms and the underlying disorder and learn about available treatments at the same time that a provider reinforces effective coping strategies (COPE Guidelines, 2011; Williams, 2014). Recommended psychoeducational topics that are beneficial to address with mothers are information about the perinatal mood or anxiety disorder, risk factors for mental illness, benefits of early treatment, discussion of treatment possibilities as well as progression/disposition (Cope Guidelines, 2011; Williams, 2014). Psychoeducation can help improve a new mother's sense of parenting competence and confidence.

Table 7.2 Treatment Modalities

Treatment Modality	*Explanation*
Self-care and Home Therapies	Self-care techniques; psychoeducation; CAM; massage, yoga, placental encapsulation
Individual Psychotherapy	Proven therapies include interpersonal therapy, cognitive therapies, psychoanalytic therapy; limited to AD only in military facilities
Pharmacotherapy	Medications including antidepressants, mood stabilizers or antipsychotics. Studies have shown many women prefer non-medication treatments and perceive medication as "giving up."
Community Support: Network	MOPS international; PSI support groups in community; PSI international warm-line
Partner or Dyadic Therapies	Marriage therapies and parent–infant therapies not generally available to military. Referred to network or obtains marital counseling from chaplains
Home-health therapies	Home-visiting programs such as New Parents support/civilian equivalent. NPSP is the only model available to military families.
Group therapies	Found to be overall beneficial in civilian communities. Usually consist of support groups/education groups. Only group study in military is Mothers in Transition Program at Camp Pendleton. Two studies presented at APA conference on postpartum support group or mother–infant group therapy
Parent–Infant Therapies	Mother–infant therapy, usually in conjunction with visit to therapist. NPSP has parent–child interaction therapy.

Self-Care

New mothers often neglect their own health, frequently neglect their own health and self-care, and are consumed with caring for their infant as well as visiting family members (Williams, 2014). Self-care basics focus on making positive changes in one's life. British Columbia Perinatal Treatment Guidelines use an acronym called *NEST-S* to help women remember the primary components of self-care. "N" is for *nutrition* and represents the importance of nutritious and healthy food in the postpartum period. In postpartum period, new mothers may struggle with finding and preparing healthy foods and may only briefly snack between feedings (Williams, 2014). Nutritional interventions can include identifying quick and healthy meal choices, learning how to eat a healthy diet, and supplementing with folic acid and vitamin D (Leung & Kaplan, 2009; Taveras et al., 2011). "E" is for *exercise* in recognition that moderate aerobic exercise can improve mood, energy and overall wellness (Daley, Macarthur, & Winter, 2007). Yoga is one sub-type of exercise that has been found to reduce prenatal and postpartum anxiety and has been routinely included in prenatal exercise programs (Buttner, Brock, O'Hara, & Stuart, 2015). "S" in the acronym stands for *sleep* to help new mothers understand the importance of adequate sleep and discuss how to help themselves obtain adequate sleep despite challenging new parent responsibilities. New mothers frequently feel sleep deprived and must learn different techniques; such mothers are usually encouraged to try to sleep when able. Sleep deprivation is associated with depression, fatigue and can mimic symptoms of depression. In severe cases, extreme sleep deprivation can trigger mania or psychotic symptoms (Goyal, Gay, & Kathryn, 2009; Lawson, Murphy, Sloan, Uleryk, & Dalfen, 2015). "T" is for *time for self* to remind mothers to set aside time for themselves by engaging in pleasurable activities that reduce stress, that mothers enjoy, and activities that give her a break from her parenting role (Williams, 2014). "S" is for *support* in recognition that a health support network can help a new mother transition to motherhood. Social support may help mothers in learning self-care activities such as meditation, relaxation, biofeedback, hypnosis, guided imagery and prayer (Williams, 2014).

Social Support

Social support in the perinatal period emphasizes the need for strong support networks (Field, Diego, Delgado, Medina, 2013; Honikman, 2008). Depressed and anxious new mothers may feel dejected and believe they have "character deficit," or are not good mothers. Social support groups during pregnancy and postpartum period create opportunities for new mothers to meet with other women who are struggling with similar challenges and allow mothers to realize they are not alone in their experience (Honikman, 2008). Social support groups create a time and place for new mothers to come together and learn from one another, create opportunities for interpersonal and social learning, and instill hope (Honikman, 2008). New group members become inspired when they hear "survivor" stories of women in who have struggled with perinatal mood and anxiety disorder, yet recovered. Further exploration of social support in civilian and military communities will occur in Chapter 12.

Individual Psychotherapies

Individual psychotherapy is a crucial component in prevention, treatment and recovery from perinatal mood disorders. Basic therapeutic principles are the installation of hope, universality, imparting information, empathic validation, therapeutic alliance, collaboration, mutuality and, potentially, a corrective emotional experience (Yalom & Leszcz, 2005). The installation of hope is crucial in any form of therapy. Women with perinatal mood and anxiety disorders often struggle with feelings of hopelessness, and feel tired, depleted, defeated and view themselves as a "bad" mother (Kleiman, 2009).

Individual psychotherapy has many different treatment approaches, often dependent on the therapeutic target. Psychotherapy treatment goals can address cognitive, emotional, behavioral and interpersonal challenges that contribute to various aspects of perinatal mood and anxiety disorders (COPE Guidelines, 2011; NICE Guidelines, 2014; Williams, 2014). The type of therapy provided is dependent on choice of the treatment provider and the needs of the patient. Both Cognitive Behavioral Therapy (CBT) and Interpersonal Therapy (IPT) are two of the most well-studied treatment modalities and have proven efficacy in treating women with mood and anxiety disorders (COPE Guidelines, 2011; NICE Guidelines, 2014; Williams, 2014). CBT and IPT are well-known treatment modalities in the therapy community and are well known to many therapists within the Military Health System.

Supportive Therapy

Supportive therapy is one of the most fundamental psychotherapies and focuses on improving a patient's sense of efficacy, confidence, hope and self-regard, self-control and adaptive skills (Winston & Goldstein, 2009). Supportive therapy offers nurturance, improved relatedness, organized feedback, attunement and reflective functioning (Markowitz, 2014; Winston & Goldstein, 2009). Supportive therapy is frequently intertwined with CBT and interpersonal therapies, and many therapists do not limit themselves to single treatment modality.

Cognitive Behavioral Therapy (CBT)

Cognitive Behavioral Therapy is a widely applicable, evidence-based treatment used to treat a variety of disorders (NICE Guidelines, 2014). Many therapists and providers inside and outside the military health system will utilize CBT. CBT has been proven effective treating mild to moderate perinatal depression and anxiety disorders (COPE Guidelines, 2011; Williams, 2014). CBT is used to treat a variety of perinatal mood and anxiety disorders with a reported success rate of 52% to 97% (COPE Guidelines, 2011; Williams, 2014). CBT therapists assist their patients in identifying automatic negative thoughts then coach their patient on how to appraise the validity of these automatic thoughts. Automatic thoughts are individual cognitions that flow rapidly in a stream of everyday consciousness and may not be accurate, relevant or rational (Wright, 2006). CBT educates patient on how automatic thoughts influence behavior, emotions and physiological changes (Bermudes, Wright, & Casey, 2009; Stuart & Koleva, 2014). See Table 7.3.

Automatic thoughts in perinatal depressive disorders center on feelings of inadequacy and doubt. For example, depressed mothers may feel overwhelmed in their struggle with interpreting their babies' signals, and internalize this struggle to develop belief that they are a "bad" mother. In contrast, automatic thoughts in perinatal anxiety disorders center on an overestimation of risk in situations and underestimate the ability to cope (Wright, 2006). For example, automatic

Table 7.3 Cognitive Behavioral Therapy Principles

1	Identify upsetting, negative distorted thoughts and assumptions
2	Understand how negative, distorted thoughts influence mood/behavior
3	Challenge and replace negative thoughts/assumptions with more realistic thoughts/ assumptions
4	Reduce behaviors that contribute to anxiety and depression
5	Increased behaviors that improve physical and mental well-being
6	Prevent and monitor for relapse
7	Lessen severity of symptoms

thoughts in anxious mother include persistent worry about the health of the infant, excessive attention to breathing patterns wherein every little variance can be interpreted as a pathological disorder.

The overarching goal in CBT is reduction in depression and anxiety symptoms and improved coping skills in order to restore the client to her previous level of functioning in a brief amount of time (Carta et al., 2015). The therapist supports the client in creating, and achieving, specific goals set by the client. Common intervention tools include but are not limited to journaling, behavior logs, role-play, "assignments" to practice skills outside of therapy, relaxation training and assertiveness training. Studies show long-lasting results from this type of therapy (Sockol, 2015).

There are many clinician resources available to help with providing CBT. British Columbia Reproductive Mental health program has two patient self-treatment manuals that patients can use or use in conjunction with a therapist. These manuals are *Coping with Depression during Pregnancy and Following the Birth* and *Coping with Anxiety during Pregnancy and Following the Birth* at www.reproductivementalhealth.ca/resources (Haring, Bodnar, Misri, Little, & Ryan, 2013; Haring, Smith, Bodnar, & Ryan, 2011; Williams, 2014). They provide practical information on depression and anxiety in the perinatal period and have exercises and activities for women to help lead to behavioral and cognitive changes (Williams, 2014).

Dialectic Behavior Therapy (DBT)

Dialectical Behavior Therapy is a subset of cognitive-based therapy that focuses on distress tolerance, mindfulness, emotional regulation and interpersonal skills (Stone, 2008; Wheelis, 2009). DBT was initially created to work with individuals with Borderline Personality Disorder—a disorder characterized by an inability to regulate emotion (Wheelis, 2009). DBT concepts have expanded beyond treatment of Borderline Personality Disorder and can be adapted to include individuals who have problems with emotional regulation and affective lability who may not carry the Borderline Personality Disorder diagnosis (Wheelis, 2009). See Table 7.4.

Table 7.4 Dialectic Behavioral Therapy Principles

Distress Tolerance	*Emotional Regulation Skills*
strengthens resiliency, which helps clients respond to painful events in a softer way.	improve feelings recognition and allow a client to observe their feelings without becoming overwhelmed by them. The client experiences a greater sense of control over their emotions, while behaving in a less reactive or destructive way.
Interpersonal Effectiveness	*Mindfulness*
provides practical tools for expressing one's beliefs and needs, limit-setting and negotiating, all while respecting others and protecting relationships.	is the practice of focusing on the present moment, as opposed to worrying about the past or the future. It also allows the client to overcome automatic negative thoughts or judgments about themselves or others.

DBT is especially effective with clients who were either born with a predisposition for intense emotions or for those who experienced early childhood trauma affecting emotional hardwiring (McKay, Wood, & Brantley, 2007; Wheelis, 2009). These individuals frequently struggle with affective lability, feelings of emptiness, and intense displays of anger (Wheelis, 2009). These behaviors cause problems in interpersonal relationships and are often outside the awareness of the individual. Individuals with difficulty regulating emotion and distress may have a history of poor attachment. As discussed in Chapter 3 on infant mental health, individuals with anxious-avoidant attachment may feel they have to minimize their emotional distress to please their caregiver and prevent a caregiver from leaving (Slade, Cohen, Sadler, & Miller, 2009).

Psychodynamic Psychotherapy

Psychodynamic psychotherapy (PDT) is a form of insight-oriented therapy wherein a therapist helps a patient examine how his or her early relationships and experiences influence the way she feels about herself and relates to others (Menken, 2008; Shelder, 2010; Williams, 2014). While PDT is used in the general population, it has not been proven effective in the literature, in part due to a difficulty of conducting PDT in a research setting (COPE Guidelines, 2011; Williams, 2014). Psychodynamic therapy may require additional training to utilize this psychotherapy and requires a different skill set than basic psychotherapies (see Table 7.5).

In the treatment of perinatal mood and anxiety disorder, PDT requires the therapist to assist a mother in exploring her entire experience of her transition

Table 7.5 Psychodynamic Therapy Concepts

Principle	*Therapist–Mother Example Interactions*
The therapeutic relationship	Sitting with a new mother and infant and exploring her experience of motherhood.
Explorations of emotions and distressful thoughts/feelings	When a mother would appear anxious/distressed when interacting with infant, she would explore meaning of the feelings.
Exploration of past relationships and current interpersonal relationships	Explore a patient's relationship with her mother and how a patient's experience being mothered influences her concept of what it meant to be a mother as well as the fear of "becoming like her mother"
Identification of recurring themes and patterns	Discuss patterns of avoiding expressing painful emotions due to fear of being rejected by attachment figure.
Discussion of unconscious childhood wish/fantasies	Discuss letting go of the childhood wish that her mother would be the "good and nurturing" mother that she did not have and be able to acknowledge that her mother did not serve as a "good" mother.

to motherhood, including feelings about conception, memories from the past and wishes from childhood (Menken, 2008). The goal of PDT is to increase self-awareness and to understand how the past affects one's present experience (Gabbard, 2009; Williams, 2014). PDT requires exploration of unconscious behaviors and cognition that are outside a mother's awareness, usually as a means to serve as a psychological defense or coping strategy (Fonagy & Target, 2009). Most forms of PDT are brief and assist a new mother in discovering unconscious processes as they manifest in current behavior (Williams, 2014).

Interpersonal Therapy (IPT)

Interpersonal Therapy focuses on role transitions such as changing roles/relationships with other people (COPE Guidelines, 2011; Williams, 2014). Thus, IPT is an ideal therapy because the transition to motherhood involves accepting new social roles and readjusting pre-existing roles (Miniati, 2014).

IPT is effective in reducing depressive symptoms in perinatal mood and anxiety disorders and has proven efficacy in research studies (Williams, 2014). IPT explores current and past relationships, interpersonal patterns in relationships, beliefs and expectations regarding role and associated affective experience (Ravitz & Watson, 2014; Spinelli, 2008). Treatment goals in IPT include alleviating interpersonal distress, analyzing role transitions/role disputes and assisting with building or making better use of social supports (Ravitz & Watson, 2014).

Specific to perinatal mood and anxiety disorder, IPT can allow a pregnant or postpartum mother analyze patterns in interpersonal relationships and discuss changes in these interpersonal roles and role transitions. In postpartum depression, women may feel they lose their identity and sense of self (Beck, 2006) and have to learn how to understand their role in society, family and accept the parental role (Spinelli, 2008). Role disputes look at a concept that in many relationships, two people have conflicting expectations about roles and expectations (Spinelli, 2008), in the midst of conflict with significant individuals in one's life (Grigoriadis & Ravitz, 2007).

Partner and Dyadic Therapies

Partner and Conjoint Therapies

Partner and conjoint therapies are psychotherapies that have purpose in addressing individual symptoms as well as addressing challenges in the marital dyad (Williams, 2014). Conjoint Psychotherapy operates on the premise that perinatal mood and anxiety disorder can cause relationship strain, especially within the couple relationship (Brandon et al., 2012; Carter, Grigoriadis, & Ross, 2010).

Partner psychotherapies consider the couple/marital relationship and view healthy partners as a potential resource with social support value (Brandon et al., 2012). Many of these partner-based dyadic therapies are modeled after IPT principles are structured similar to individual interpersonal therapy concepts (Carter et al., 2010). See Table 7.6.

Perinatal dyadic therapy is designed to reduce an individual's depressive symptoms while simultaneously also improving the quality of a couple's relationships (Carter et al., 2010). Similar to individual IPT, a therapist assists the couple in identifying possible ways each member may contribute to the resolution of the dispute and discuss strategies to improve communication and shifting expectations (Carter et al., 2010).

Table 7.6 Partner-Assisted Therapy Concepts

Partner-assisted therapies
• Identify the existing maternal and paternal stressors • Identify dyadic expectations each hold around roles as mother or father • Uncover core emotions around the stressors and expectations, exploring the realities and modifying appraisals • Enlist the partner in accepting the woman's feelings and responding in a "language" that she finds supportive • Assessing couple's interactions, illuminating negativity and experimenting with more positive interchanges • Increase the partner's emotional and instrumental support, thereby reducing the maternal stressors

Parent–Infant Dyadic Therapies

While individually based psychotherapies are proven to be effective in treating mothers with perinatal mood and anxiety disorders, therapies only involving the mother are not associated with better child outcomes or improvements in a mother–infant relationship in the long term (Paris, Spielman, & Bolton, 2009). Functional sleep, feeding and behavioral disorders are some of the most frequent reasons for psychiatric consultation for children under 3 years old (COPE Guidelines, 2011; Williams, 2014). Parent–infant therapy has been proven in research studies to improve a child/infant's symptoms, mother–infant interaction, maternal self-esteem/confidence, decrease parenting stress, and reduce mother–infant conflict (Williams, 2014)

The field of infant mental health has led to the creation of parent–infant dyadic therapies. Parent–infant psychotherapy is a therapeutic intervention that aims to improve the quality of parent-infant interaction and social-emotional functioning of the baby (Williams, 2014). For simplicity purposes, we will use the term "mother–infant" therapies, while recognizing that if therapy may be father–infant therapies or triadic therapy (Williams, 2014). The primary goal of mother–infant therapy is to improve the quality of a mother's relationship with her infant and increase her ability to remain affectively present in interactions with her infant (Paris et al., 2009). Mother–infant therapy focuses on the history of the mother (especially her attachment experience), mother–baby connections during pregnancy, and observable and deducible parent–child interactional experience (Williams, 2014). Selma Freiberg was one of the founders of mother–infant therapy through her describing the concept of transgenerational transmission of attachment disorders (Frailberg, Adelson, & Shapiro, 1975). Subsequent research has added to the idea of transgenerational transmission of attachment by identifying the notion of a corrective emotional experience; positive parenting experiences elicited with the help of therapist can serve as corrective experiences to help mother/parent move past prior childhood trauma (Guedeney, Guedeney, Wendland, & Burtchen, 2014; Lieberman & Van Horn, 2013).

In mother–infant psychotherapy, the presence of the infant is used to catalyze change throughout the therapeutic process (Paris et al., 2009). A mother–infant therapist observes and attends to the infant's actions and communications in the "here and now" and can create connections between maternal experience and infant behavior (Paris et al., 2009).

A therapist needs to be closely attuned to the infant's emotional state and assist the parent in understanding the meaning of an infant's communication, as well as close attunement to the parent's emotional state (Weatherston, 2000). As an outside observer, a therapist has a chance to observe two patients: the parent and the infant. As an outside observer, a therapist engaging in mother–infant therapy can notice subtle emotional changes that a parent may not be aware of, such as the way a parent handles his or her baby when frustrated or the shift of

Table 7.7 Mother–Infant Therapy Concepts

Parent–infant therapy core beliefs (Weatherston, 2000)
• Optimal growth and development occur within nurturing relationships • The birth and care of a baby offer a family the possibility of new relationships, growth and change • What happens in the early years affects the course of development across the lifespan • Early developing attachment relationships may be distorted or disturbed by parental histories of unresolved trauma and losses • The therapeutic process of a parent–infant therapy may reduce the risk of relationship failure and offer the hopefulness of warm and nurturing parenting responses

a parent's affect (or lack thereof) in response to infant emotional expression. The therapist may then "wonder aloud" about his or her observations of parent mood and inquire what a parent may be experiencing (Weatherston, 2000). See Table 7.7.

When working with a mother during mother–infant psychotherapy, a therapist must develop a rapport that creates a "holding environment" in which a mother feels safe and secure to express a variety of emotions as well as discussed stories of present/recent relationships. A mother may disclose past stories of trauma from her childhood and disrupted relationships between herself and her mother (Paris et al., 2009). While listening to a mother, a therapist concurrently watches the infant to discover clues as to what may be going on in the mother–infant dyad (Weatherston, 2000). For instance, a mother may see herself in her infant, and be reminded of her past. By understanding a mother's history of relationships and care, a therapist will understand her ability or inability to nurture and protect her child (Weatherston, 2000).

Group Therapies

Despite its benefits, group therapy is often an underappreciated therapy and treatment modality. While individual studies have stronger evidence of efficacy than group therapies, there is still empiric evidence affirming the benefits of group therapy (Goodman & Santangelo, 2011; Klier, Muzik, Rosenblum, & Lenz, 2001). Group therapy provides a safe and accepting place to vent frustration and fears, and serves as a means to receive comfort and encouragement from other moms (COPE Guidelines, 2011; Williams, 2014). In non-perinatal populations, group therapy has been shown to be at least equal to individual psychotherapy in its power to provide meaningful benefits (Yalom & Leszcz, 2005).

Yalom identifies seven core therapeutic factors: instillation of hope, universality, imparting information, altruism, a corrective recapitulation of the primary family group, development of social techniques, and imitative behavior

(Yalom & Leszcz, 2005). Universality describes the concept of normalizing one's experience and realizing he or she is not alone. In group therapy, group members discover that they are not alone in their experience; other mothers often experience similar challenges (Yalom & Leszcz, 2005). Group therapy also allows for the use of altruism because it provides a client with an opportunity to help others (Yalom & Leszcz, 2005). Group therapy also builds off principles of social learning as individuals can learn from one another. In a group of perinatal mood and anxiety disorders, this becomes a critical source of support as mothers learn they are not alone and that many other mothers are sharing in a similar experience.

The group can reduce social isolation, facilitate mutual emotional support, foster a sense of altruism, provide an avenue for interpersonal learning and emphasize the commonality of postpartum distress. Many techniques of group therapy are constructed from individual psychotherapy principles. For instance, IPT-based group therapy built off the known efficacy that individualized IPT therapy has for the interpersonal difficulties /role transition that is associated with motherhood (Klier et al., 2001).

A unique group therapy modality is constructed off concepts of mother–infant group therapy (Clark, Tluczek, & Brown, 2008). Group psychodynamic therapy examines interpersonal relationships that develop within the group with the belief that interpersonal difficulties in an individual's life will manifest themselves in the group milieu (Yalom & Leszcz, 2005).

In addition to addressing interpersonal difficulties that manifest in the group, mother–infant therapy specifically addresses the mother–infant attachment/bond, which is specifically relevant to postpartum depression.

Mother–infant group therapy (M-ITG) addresses social isolation and lack of emotional support that is often associated with postpartum depression. Additinally, M-ITG offers mothers an ability to understand how depression affects them as well as how it interpersonally relates to others (Clark et al., 2008). Specifically, this M-ITG allows mothers to learn better ways of relating/coping, which will then theoretically enable them to be more available to their infants (Clark et al., 2008). In Clark et al.'s study, mothers and infants met concurrently for 90 minutes each, followed by a final 30 minutes of examining the mother–infant relationship (also referred to as a dyad). The mother's group utilized psychodynamic strategies that assisted mothers in exploring early relationship histories and the impact of these prior experiences on current emotional experiences/interpersonal relationships. Mothers were encouraged to explore problematic relationships, clarify the nature of relationship difficulties, analyze their communication style and then use the therapeutic environment to lead to behavioral change (Clark et al., 2008). See Table 7.8.

The group format specifically benefited new mothers by reducing social isolation, facilitating emotional support, fostering a sense of altruism, and providing interpersonal learning and validation of common postpartum experiences (Clark et al., 2008; Yalom, 2005). The treatment focused on enabling

Table 7.8 Mother–Infant Group Therapy Principles (Clark et al., 2008)

- Ameliorate the mother's depressive symptoms
- Address the mother's intrapsychic conflicts related to her own experiences of being parented
- Reduce the mother's social isolation
- Provide an emotionally responsive environment for the infant that supports his or her development
- Facilitate positive mother–infant interactions
- Enhance the quality of the mother's relationship with her partner, including communication/problem-solving capacities of both as well as improve the mother's overall functioning both within and outside her family

mothers to recognize interpersonal, intrapsychic and cognitive patterns that contributed to depressive symptoms; developed strategies and coping mechanisms for reducing depressive symptoms; participated in the group process, enabling them to broaden social support/reduce social isolations; increased mother's awareness of her own needs and enhanced a mother's ability to fulfill her needs as well as needs of her infant and increased a mother's ability to empathetically care for her infant (Clark et al., 2008). Overall, study results were positive, showing significant improvement in both maternal depression and improvement of mother–child interaction and are unique in that they offer clinicians the ability to treat relationships instead of just depression.

Due to the cost-effectiveness of the group, group therapy is a model being embraced by the military and has an opportunity for expansion (Reay et al., 2013). Such concepts will be explored in the discussion of two military treatments/intervention models in Chapter 11.

Summary

As one can see, many different non-pharmacological treatment modalities are evidence-based for women with perinatal mood and anxiety disorder, and most of these are available to military service members either in the military health system or the TRICARE network. Lack of treatment has untold consequences for a mother, infant and family. It is our goal to familiarize providers and patients with these therapies, as they are feasible in most environments including military settings. In the next chapter, we will tackle the complicated topic of psychopharmacological and somatic therapy treatment modalities.

References

Beck, C. T. (2006). Postpartum depression: It isn't just the blues. *American Journal of Nursing, 106*(5), 40–50; quiz 50–41.

Bermudes, R., Wright, J., & Casey, D. (2009). Techniques of cognitive behavioral therapy. In G. Gabbard (Ed.), *Textbook of Psychotherapeutic Treatments* [E-Reader Version]. Arlington, VA: American Psychiatric Publishing, Inc.

BeyondBlue. (2011). Clinical Practice Guidelines (COPE): Depression and Related Disorders—Anxiety, Bipolar Disorder and Puerperal Psychosis—in the Perinatal Period: A Guideline for Primary Care Health Professionals. Australian Government: National Health and Medical Research Counsel. Retrieved from www.beyondblue.org.au

Brandon, A. R., Ceccotti, N., Hynan, L. S., Shivakumar, G., Johnson, N., & Jarrett, R. B. (2012). Proof of concept: Partner-assisted interpersonal psychotherapy for perinatal depression. *Archives of Women's Mental Health, 15*(6), 469–480. doi:10.1007/s00737–012–0311–1

Buttner, M., Brock, R., O'Hara, M., & Stuart, S. (2015). Efficacy of yoga for depressed postpartum women: A randomized controlled trial. *Complementary Therapies in Clinical Practice, 21*, 94–100.

Carta, G., D'Alfonso, A., Parisse, V., Di Fonso, A., Casacchia, M., & Patacchiola, F. (2015). How does early cognitive behavioral therapy reduce postpartum depression? *Clinical and Experimental Obstetrics & Gynecology, 42*(1), 49–52. https://www.ncbi.nlm.nih.gov/pubmed/25864281

Carter, W., Grigoriadis, S., & Ross, L. (2010). Relationship distress and depression in postpartum women: Literature review and introduction of a conjoint interpersonal psychotherapy intervention. *Archives of Women's Mental Health, 13*, 279–284. doi:10.1007/s00737–009–0136–8

Clark, R., Tluczek, A., & Brown, R. (2008). A mother-infant therapy group model for postpartum depression. *Infant Mental Health Journal, 29*(5), 514–536. doi:10.1002/imhj.20189

Collins, C., & MacDermid-Wadsworth, S. (2014). Understanding military families: Their characteristics, strengths, and challenges. In S. Cozza, M. Goldenberg, & R. Ursano (Eds.), *Care of Military Service Members, Veterans, and Their Families* [E-Readers Version]. Arlington, VA: American Psychiatric Publishing, Inc. http://dx.doi.org/10.1176/appi.books.9781585625161.sc02

Daley, A. J., Macarthur, C., & Winter, H. (2007). The role of exercise in treating postpartum depression: A review of the literature. *Journal of Midwifery & Women's Health, 52*(1), 56–62. doi:10.1016/j.jmwh.2006.08.017

Field, T., Diego, M., Delgado, J., & Medina, L. (2013). Peer support and interpersonal psychotherapy groups experienced decreased prenatal depression, anxiety and cortisol. *Early Human Development, 89*, 621–614.

Fonagy, P., & Target, M. (2009). Theoretical models of psychodynamic psychotherapy. In G. Gabbard (Ed.), *Textbook of Psychotherapeutic Treatments*. Arlington, VA: American Psychiatric Publishing, Inc. Retrieved from http://dx.doi.org/10.1176/appi.books.9781585623648.gg01

Frailberg, S., Adelson, E., & Shapiro, V. (1975). Ghosts in the nursery: A psychoanalytic approach to the problems of impaired infant-mother relationships. *The American Journal of Child Psychiatry, 14*(1–4), 387–421.

Gabbard, G. (2009). Techniques of psychodynamic psychotherapy. In G. Gabbard (Ed.), *Textbook of Psychotherapeutic Treatments* (pp. 42–132). Washington, DC: American Psychiatric Publishing, Inc.

Goodman, J. (2009). Women's attitudes, preferences, and perceived barriers to treatment for perinatal depression. *Birth, 36*(1), 60.

Goodman, S. H., Broth, M. R., Hall, C. M., & Stowe, Z. N. (2008). Treatment of postpartum depression in mothers: Secondary benefits to the infants. *Infant Mental Health Journal, 29*(5), 492–513.

Goodman, J., & Santangelo, G. (2011). Group treatment for postpartum depression: A systematic review. *Arch Womens Ment Health, 14*, 277–293. doi:10.1007/s00737–011–0225–3

Goyal, D., Gay, C., & Kathryn, L. (2009). Fragmented maternal sleep is more strongly correlated with depressive symptoms than infant temperament at three months postpartum. *Archives of Women's Mental Health, 12*, 229–237.

Grigoriadis, S., & Ravitz, P. (2007). An approach to interpersonal psychotherapy for postpartum depression. *Canadian Family Physician, 53* (September), 1469–1475. Retrieved from https://www.ncbi.nlm.nih.gov/pubmed/17872875

Guedeney, A., Guedeney, N., Wendland, J., & Burtchen, N. (2014). Treatment—mother–infant relationship psychotherapy. *Best Practice & Research Clinical Obstetrics and Gynaecology, 28*, 135–145.

Haring, M., Bodnar, D., Misri, S., Little, R., & Ryan, D. (2013). *Coping with Anxiety during Pregnancy and Following the Birth: A Cognitive Behavior Therapy-Based Self Management Guide for Women and Healthcare Providers*. British Columbia. Retrieved from www.bcmhas.ca

Haring, M., Smith, J., Bodnar, D., & Ryan, D. (2011). *Coping with Depression during Pregnancy and Following the Birth: A Cognitive Behavior Therapy Based Self-Management*. BC Mental Health and Addiction Services, British Columbia. Retrieved from www.bcmhas.ca

Honikman, J. (2008). The role of social support in the prevention, intervention, and treatment of perinatal mood disorders. In S. Stone & A. Menken (Eds.), *Perinatal and Postpartum Mood Disorders: Perspectives and Treatment Guide for the Health Care Practitioner* [E-Reader Version]. New York: Springer.

Johnson, P., Knauss, L., Faran, M., & Ban, P. (2014). Military children & programs that meet their needs. In S. Cozza, M. Goldenberg, & R. Ursano (Eds.), *Care of Military Service Members, Veterans, and Their Families* [E-Reader Version]. Arlington, VA: American Psychiatric Publishing, Inc. Retrieved from http://dx.doi.org/10.1176/appi.books.9781585625161.sc03

Kleiman, K. (2009). *Therapy and the Postpartum Woman: Notes on Healing Postpartum Depression for Clinicians and the Women Who Seek Their Help*. New York: Routledge Taylor&Francis.

Klier, C., Muzik, M., Rosenblum, K., & Lenz, G. (2001). Interpersonal Psychotherapy adapted for the group setting in the treatment of postpartum depression. *The Journal of Psychotherapy Practice and Research, 10*(2), 124–131.

Lawson, A., Murphy, K., Sloan, E., Uleryk, E., & Dalfen, A. (2015). The relationship between sleep and postpartum mental disorders: A systematic review. *Journal of Affective Disorders, 176*, 65–77.

Leung, B. M., & Kaplan, B. J. (2009). Perinatal depression: Prevalence, risks, and the nutrition link—a review of the literature. *Journal of American Dietetic Association, 109*(9), 1566–1575. doi:10.1016/j.jada.2009.06.368

Lieberman, A., & Van Horn, P. (2013). Infants and young children in military families: A conceptual model for change. *Clinical Child and Family Psychology Review, 16*, 282–293.

Markowitz, J. (2014). What is supportive psychotherapy? *FOCUS: The Journal of Lifelong Learning in Psychiatry, 12*(3), 285–289.

McKay, M., Wood, J. C., & Brantley, J. (2007). *The Dialectical Behavior Therapy Skills Workbook: Practical DBT Exercises for Learning Mindfulness, Interpersonal Effectiveness, Emotion Regulation & Distress Tolerance*. Oakland, CA: New Harbinger Publications.

Menken, A. (2008). A psychodynamic approach to treatment for postpartum depression. In S. Stone & A. Menken (Eds.), *Perinatal and Postpartum Mood Disorders: Perspectives and Treatment Guide for the Health Care Practitioner* [E-Reader Version]. New York: Springer.

Miniati, M., Callari, A., Calugi, S., Rucci, P., Savino, M., Mauri, M., & Dell'Osso, L. (2014). Interpersonal psychotherapy for postpartum depression: A systematic review. *Archves of Women's Mental Health, 17*(4), 257–268. doi:10.1007/s00737–014–0442–7

National Institute of Health and Care Excellence (NICE). (2014). Antenatal and postnatal mental health: Clinical management and service guideline. *Clinical Guideline.* Retrieved from www.Nice.org.uk/guidance/cg192

O'Mahen, H., & Flynn, H. (2008). Preferences and perceived barriers to treatment for depression during the perinatal period. *Journal of Women's Health, 17*(8), 1301–1309. doi: 10.1089/jwh.2007.0631.

Paris, R., Spielman, E., & Bolton, R. E. (2009). Mother-infant psychotherapy: Examining the therapeutic process of change. *Infant Mental Health Journal, 30*(3), 301–319. doi:10.1002/imhj.20216

Ravitz, P., & Watson, P. (2014). Interpersonal psychotherapy: Healing with a relational focus. *FOCUS: The Journal of Lifelong Learning in Psychiatry, 12*(3), 275.

Reay, R. E., Owen, C., Shadbolt, B., Raphael, B., Mulcahy, R., & Wilkinson, R. B. (2013). Trajectories of long-term outcomes for postnatally depressed mothers treated with group interpersonal psychotherapy. *Archives of Women's Mental Health, 15*, 217–228. doi:10.1007/s00737–012–0280–4

Shelder, J. (2010). The efficacy of psychodynamic psychotherapy. *American Psychologist, 65*(2), 98–109.

Slade, A., Cohen, L., Sadler, L., & Miller, M. (2009). The psychology and psychopathology of pregnancy. In C. Zeanah (Ed.), *Handbook of Infant Mental Health* (3rd ed., Ch. 5, pp. 80–103). New York: The Guilford Press.

Sockol, L. E. (2015). A systematic review of the efficacy of cognitive behavioral therapy for treating and preventing perinatal depression. *Journal of Affect Disorders, 177*, 7–21. doi:10.1016/j.jad.2015.01.052

Spinelli, M. (2008). Treating antepartum depression: Interpersonal therapy. In S. Stone & A. Menken (Eds.), *Perinatal and Postpartum Mood Disorders* [E-Reader Version]. New York: Springer.

Stone, S. (2008). Comorbid presentation in perinatal mental health: Dialectic behavioral therapy as a treatment model. In S. Stone & A. Menken (Eds.), *Perinatal and Postpartum Mood Disorders: Perspective and Treatment Guide for the Health Care Practitioner* [E-Reader Version]. New York: Springer.

Stuart, S., & Koleva, H. (2014). Psychological treatments for perinatal depression. *Best Practice & Research Clinical Obstetrics and Gynaecology, 28*, 61–70.

Taveras, E. M., Blackburn, K., Gillman, M., Haines, J., McDonald, J., Price, S., & Oken, E. (2011). First steps for mommy and me: A pilot intervention to improve nutrition and physical activity behaviors of postpartum mothers and their infants. *Maternal Child Health, 15*(8), 1217–1227. doi:10.1007/s10995–010–0696–2

Verdeli, H., Baily, C., Vousoura, E., Belser, A., Manos, G., & Singla, D. (2011). The case for treating depression in military spouses. *Journal of Family Psychology, 25*(4), 488–496. doi:10.1037/a0024525

Weatherston, D. (2000). The Infant Mental Health Specialist. Zero to Three: National Center for Infants, Toddlers and Families (October/November).

Wheelis, J. (2009). Theory and practice of dialectic behavioral therapy. In G. Gabbard (Ed.), *Textbook of Psychotherapeutic Treatments* [E-Reader Version]. Arlington, VA: American Psychiatric Publishing, Inc. Retrieved from http://dx.doi.org/10.1176/appi.books.9781585623648.gg27

Williams, J. (2014). Best practice guidelines for mental health disorders in the perinatal period. *BC Mental Health.* Retrieved from http://www.perinatalservicesbc.ca/health-professionals/guidelines-standards/maternal (Accessed on 24 January, 2016).

Winston, A., & Goldstein, M. (2009). Theory of supportive psychotherapy. In G. Gabbard (Ed.), *Textbook of Psychotherapeutic Treatments* [E-Reader Version]. Arlington, VA: American Psychiatric Publishing, Inc. Retrieved from http://dx.doi.org/10.1176/appi.books.9781585623648.gg14

Wright, J. (2006). Cognitive behavior therapy: Basic principles and recent advances. *FOCUS: The Journal of Lifelong Learning in Psychiatry, 4*(2), 123–177.

Yalom, I., & Leszcz, M. (2005). *The Theory and Practice of Group Psychotherapy* (5th ed.). New York, NY: Basic Books.

Yonkers, K., Wisner, K., Stewart, D., Oberlander, T., Dell, D., Stotland, N., . . . Lockwood, C. (2012). The management of depression during pregnancy: A report from the American Psychiatric Association and the American College of obstetricians and gynecologists. *FOCUS: The Journal of Lifelong Learning in Psychiatry, 10*(1), 78–89.

Chapter 8

Pharmacological and Somatic Treatments in the Perinatal Period

Melinda A. Thiam, Carla W. Schnitzlein, David S. Hodson, and Daniel J. Lee

Important Caveats for this Chapter

Data involving pregnant women is largely limited to case reports, case series and/or post-marketing surveillance (COPE Guidelines, 2011; www.womensmentalhealth.org). For many psychoactive medications, determination of potential teratogenicity is made from small cohorts of several hundred women or less (Ray & Stowe, 2014; www.womensmentalhealth.org). While the U.S. Food and Drug Association (FDA) assigns each medication a class based upon potential teratogenicity, these classes should be seen as a useful starting point during informed consent rather than an absolute determination of suitability in pregnancy (www.infantrisk.org). Providers should consider the risks versus benefits of each medication as well as consider a patient's preference. This chapter is *not* a complete guide to care. Instead, this chapter should serve to assist providers in understanding the current evidenced-based research on various medications. Treatment should be specific to an individual patient; approaches may differ dependent on clinical context. Additionally, the field of medicine is perpetually changing; new evidence may be published in the future that contradicts evidence available upon writing this chapter. Clinicians are encouraged to use their best clinical judgment in the treatment of pregnant and postpartum patients. While there are many additional challenges to consider in the treatment of mental disorders in pregnant women as a whole, this chapter will focus on treatment in pregnant and postpartum women who are active duty or active duty family members. Treatment challenges and potential barriers to care may present differently in general pregnant and postpartum population and may have different challenges than treatment in a military setting.

Treatment Overview

The prior chapters have emphasized how maternal mental health impacts infant and child mental health. Given such, it is well understood that medications a woman takes during pregnancy can affect her developing baby. Whenever possible, pregnant women and clinicians usually prefer to utilize non-pharmacological treatments to minimize fetal exposure to medications. However, there are times when psychotherapy/social support are not sufficient to successfully treat a mother's mental illness. Risk of medication during pregnancy is essential to understand; however, it is also important to recognize that there are risks to infant of untreated maternal illness during pregnancy and postpartum period of untreated mental illness.

Treatment Settings

Most mood and anxiety disorders are treated by primary care providers in a general setting as well as the perinatal population.(Deneke, 2015). Despite being responsible for much of the treatment of depression/anxiety disorders, primary care clinicians often complete their initial specialty training having received little to no training in the diagnosis and treatment of mental illness (Leigh, Stewart, & Mallios, 2006). Likewise, while mental health prescribers such as psychiatrists and psychiatric nurse practitioners training are proficient in treating numerous types of mental illness, they usually receive minimal exposure to reproductive psychiatry. Unfortunately, this can lead to obstetric providers referring pregnant or postpartum mothers to a behavioral health provider, just to have the behavioral health providers refer the women to her obstetrician. Both primary care and behavioral health providers may be reluctant to treat pregnant or breastfeeding mothers with mental illness due to lack of expertise, fear of lawsuit or overestimation of risk (Osborne et al., 2015).

Barriers to Care

While psychotherapy is clearly effective for many pregnant women with mild-to-moderate depression, in reality it may be difficult to obtain due to limited availability, accessibility and social acceptability (Ray & Stowe, 2014; Stowe, 2012). In the perinatal population, pharmacological treatment also is limited by both patient and clinician acceptability of treatment.

In the United States, there is limited accessibility to care by trained mental health prescribers such as psychiatrists and psychiatric nurse practitioners. Outside the perinatal period, psychiatric prescribers often have a 2- to 3-month backlog of wait times, with both primary care and the emergency room serving as the backup for emergencies. This wait time may be even longer for a pregnant patient, and often there is even more limited access to mental health clinicians who are comfortable, and willing, to prescribe medications to a pregnant patient. In the military health system, family members are often deferred to the network, and there frequently is a limited number of providers who accept TRICARE, especially in more rural areas. Similar to the general population, there may be financial constraints and occupational and/or childcare concerns that limit the ability to drive a long distance to treatment. Availability and accessibility are affected by both patient and clinician acceptability.

Clinicians may be reluctant to treat pregnant women, and they may feel obligated to defer or discontinue medication treatment when their patient becomes pregnant.

Attitudes regarding various treatments can significantly affect both selections of treatment(s) and patient compliance. For pregnant mothers, concerns about medication may be based on fear of harming their child, a desire to breastfeed following parturition and/or an internalized stigma that leads them to equate taking pharmacological treatment with character flaws and/or moral/spiritual weakness (Ray & Stowe, 2014). A pregnant woman's overestimation of risk can lead to outright rejection of medication before potential benefits can be discussed or, alternatively, noncompliance with prescribed medication after leaving a clinician's office (Goodman, 2009; Ray & Stowe, 2014).

Pharmacotherapy for Depression in the Perinatal Period

Limitations of Available Evidence

The media often permits advertisements on television that announces legal action related to medication, especially in medication in pregnancy, which then exacerbates clinical angst and concern about legal liability (Ray & Stowe, 2014). The difference between real and perceived risk is partly due to limitations of validity and reliability of medication trials in the pregnant population. Moral and ethical issues preclude the ability to conduct randomized controlled trials, which are traditionally the gold standard in evidenced-based medicine. To avoid bias, randomized controlled trial would require pregnant women to be purposely exposed to interventions with potential teratogenic effects (Ray & Stowe, 2012). Instead, drug studies related to pregnancy are limited to observation and correlation. Like most medication studies of non-pregnant adults, these trials frequently have design flaws, incomplete data reporting, and multiple forms of bias (Ray & Stowe, 2014).

As a whole, data collection in these studies is deeply flawed. Most perinatal medication exposure data are gathered via questionnaire or interviews months to years after delivery (Newport, Fernandez, Juric, & Stowe, 2014). Unfortunately, recall bias may interfere with accurate reporting beyond 6 months (Chaudron, 2013; Ray & Stowe, 2014). This time point marks the transition from accurate reporting to systematic underreporting of depression symptoms and use of non-psychoactive medication (Chaudron, 2013; Ray & Stowe, 2014).

Additionally, studies specifically involving pregnant women are typically retrospective case reports, case series and post-marketing drug surveillance (COPE Guidelines, 2011; NICE Guidelines, 2014; Yonkers et al., 2012), supplemented with research on non-human mammals (Newport et al., 2014). In the absence of prospective, randomized controlled trials, causality cannot be definitively evaluated in humans.

Many drug studies in the perinatal population are unable to confirm antidepressant exposure; instead, they rely on maternal self-report regarding drug exposure and other environment exposures (Ray & Stowe, 2014). Additionally, these studies frequently are unable to differentiate between the risk untreated maternal depression has on an infant and the reliance on maternal self-report and recall (Higgins et al., 2011; Ray & Stowe, 2014).

Many studies involving pregnant women fail to control for or exclude other medications, raising the prospect of teratogenicity from other sources (Newport et al., 2014). Differences in socio-economic/environmental factors that contribute to the incidence of mental illness are often ignored as well (Newport et al., 2014). All risk factors for mental illness, general maternal health, as well as psychosocial risk factors also increase the risk of adverse fetal outcomes, regardless of psychoactive medication status (Ray & Stowe, 2014).

Other studies involving pregnant women cite inconsistent/inadequate dosing of psychoactive medications (Chaudron, 2013; Newport et al., 2014; Ray & Stowe, 2014). As is true of many psychoactive medication studies, median dosages tend to be lower than those typically used in clinical practice, and pill counts are generally not performed to ensure compliance with prescribed medications (Newport, Ray & Stowe, Chaudron, 2013; Goodman, 2009). Even when women take antidepressants during pregnancy, almost 8% are taking doses lower than recommended (Chaudron, 2013). Studies are frequently unable to ensure compliance. At times, women in these studies reported compliance, yet their blood/urine samples had undetectable medication levels (Ray & Stowe, 2014; Stowe, 2012).

Baseline Risks: Pregnancy Risk Versus Medication Risk

Evaluation of psychoactive medication teratogenicity is complicated by the fact that some risk of birth defects exists at the baseline, and polypharmacy is common in the general population (Newport et al., 2014). Under optimal circumstances, there appears to be a 3%–4% baseline risk of the large fetal malformations in pregnancy (Newport et al., 2014). Thus, in the absence of prospective, randomized, controlled trials, baseline risk is difficult to separate from psychoactive medication risk. All medications pass through the placenta and create exposure risk to the fetus (Chaudron, 2013). Unfortunately, despite this large number of woman exposed to psychotropics in pregnancy, the data is of limited usefulness because researchers cannot definitively discern when and how long exposure occurred during pregnancy (Newport et al., 2014).

Factors to Consider When Treating Depression in Pregnancy

Discussions regarding maintenance, initiation or discontinuation of antidepressants during pregnancy require careful presentation of informed consent. While addressing risks of medication during pregnancy, it is critical to emphasize that *avoiding medication does not negate risk.* We have seen evidence of this principle in earlier chapters where we discussed the potential risks of untreated depression due to the risk of adverse outcome both for the mother, infant and mother–infant relationship.

Depression is a chronic illness that often manifests itself in a cyclical pattern with depressive episodes lasting weeks to months followed by complete or incomplete remission of symptoms for a variable period (McInnis, Riba, & Greden, 2014). Individuals with prior episodes of depression (during and/or out of the perinatal period) are at increased risk of depression during pregnancy and following parturition (Ray & Stowe, 2014). Women who discontinue their antidepressants during pregnancy are 5 times as likely to have a relapse in comparison to mothers who maintained antidepressant treatment (Chaudron, 2013; Cohen et al., 2006). Factors that clinicians should consider are the severity of current or pre-existing depressive disorder, as well as family history of severe postpartum depression in close relatives. Symptoms of more severe illness include poor function during prior depressive episode(s), prolonged duration of depressive symptoms, difficult to manage treatment-refractory, development of active suicidal ideation during previous episode(s) and previous suicide attempts or instances of self-harm (Cohen et al., 2010).

Medication Discontinuation

Upon discovering pregnancy, both patients and clinicians alike often have the first inclination to discontinue all antidepressants (Ray & Stowe, 2014). Discontinuing antidepressants occurs due to overestimation of potential harm posed by the medication along with underestimation of both mental illness severity and positive benefits derived from antidepressants. The strongest evidence statement at this time is that no correlation exists between most first-line antidepressants and adverse fetal outcomes in humans (COPE Guidelines, 2011; Newport et al., 2014; NICE Guidelines, 2014; Yonkers et al., 2012).

Discontinuation of antidepressants during pregnancy frequently correlates with increased risk of relapse (Cohen et al., 2010). The baseline rate of relapse for women with depression who maintain their antidepressant(s) is 26% (Cohen et al., 2010). This baseline rate rises to a 68% risk of relapse in the first trimester and a 90% likelihood of relapse during the second trimester if antidepressant(s) are discontinued during pregnancy (Robinson, 2012). In addition to depression relapse, 70.3% of women discontinuing antidepressant(s) had adverse outcomes with 33% becoming suicidal (Robinson, 2012).

Antidepressant Treatment in Pregnancy

Medications

Monoamine Oxidase Inhibitors (MAOIs) and Tricyclic Antidepressants (TCAs)

Two of the first antidepressant classes are tricyclic antidepressants (TCAs) and monoamine oxidase inhibitors (MAOIs). While these medication classes may be advantageous and efficient to treat depression, they also have more risks and side effects than new medication classes and are no longer used as a primary treatment for depression. We recommend that the use of these medications be limited to trained psychiatrists and thus will not discuss these two classes of medication.

Selective Serotonin Reuptake Inhibitors (SSRIs)

Upon the introduction of fluoxetine in 1986, SSRIs became first-line medications recommended for depression, anxiety disorders, OCD and trauma-related disorders (Ray & Stowe, 2014). SSRIs work by preventing reuptake of serotonin, which then assists in increasing levels of serotonin available at neuronal synapses. Because estrogen has synergistic effects on serotonin, it is hypothesized that decreases in estrogen in postpartum period lead to decreased serotonin, which can then predispose a new mother to postpartum depression (Ray & Stowe, 2014).

SSRIs are not selective to the brain and can cause side effects by affecting different body systems, particularly gastrointestinal side effects as well as sexual side effects in the adult. Given the potential side effects of medication in the mother, there will be potential side effects in the fetus during pregnancy because all drugs cross the placenta in pregnancy and can secrete into breast milk. SSRI medications include fluoxetine (Prozac), sertraline (Zoloft), escitalopram (Lexapro), citalopram (Celexa), paroxetine (Paxil) and fluvoxamine (Luvox). For the most part, the determination of which SSRI to use is usually based on prior efficacy (individual already had a positive response to medication) as well as side effects. Fluoxetine has been around the longest and thus has the greatest amount of literature/safety data. It also has the longest half-life of medication and thus in the general population can be advantageous to an individual who has a tendency to forget medications. On the other hand, the one medication that we recommend most caution is Paroxetine. Paroxetine has some greater side effects, has the shortest half-life, contributes to weight gain and has a class D rating for pregnancy due to correlation with increased risk of pulmonary hypertension that is greater than other medications in its class (Stewart & Vigod, 2014).

Selective Serotonin-Norepinephrine Reuptake Inhibitors (SNRIs)

Another class of antidepressants includes serotonin-norepinephrine reuptake inhibitors (SRNIs). The three main medications in this class include venlafaxine (Effexor), duloxetine (Cymbalta) and desvenlafaxine (Pristiq). SNRIs are also used for the treatment of depression/anxiety, usually the second choice after one considers an SSRI. SNRIs are particularly beneficial if there are much low energy/cognitive/attention problems due to depression, the noradrenergic aspects can be beneficial, while still having the presence of serotonin to target anxiety. Duloxetine is FDA approved for treatment of chronic pain, and thus pregnant women who have chronic pain may benefit from this medication. Both venlafaxine and duloxetine are also thought to be advantageous for attentions/concentration problems seen in depression/anxiety as well as ADHD and may be a safer alternative to a stimulant (Roy-Burne, 2014). There are no significant different side effects of SNRIs compared to SSRIs in pregnancy/postpartum risk except increased likelihood of preeclampsia. It is suspected that increased risk of preeclampsia may be due to effects of norepinephrine (which can increase heart rate and blood pressure). Although desvenlafaxine is newer with less data, given its similar class/chemical structure to venlafaxine, it could be conjectured that its side effects/risks should be similar. Further studies are needed, and typically desvenlafaxine is non-formulary in many health care plans.

The atypical antidepressants commonly used include bupropion (Wellbutrin), mirtazapine (Remeron) and trazodone. Bupropion acts on norepinephrine and dopamine reuptake receptors and has been preferred in atypical depression, depression with neurovegetative/neurocognitive symptoms, as well as attention/concentration disorders. Given the lack of serotonin effects, it is not beneficial for anxiety and can thus actually make anxiety worse. On the other hand, the lack of serotonin effects also means an absence of the sexual side effects that are seen in both SNRIs and SSRIs. Bupropion is also preferred by patients concerned about weight gain as it is one antidepressant that can be associated with weight loss. Mirtazapine is a lesser known antidepressant, predominately used to treat insomnia due to sedating side effects. Both Mirtazepine and Paroxetine are known to cause weight gain. Like Mirtazepine, Trazodone is commonly used as a sleep aid, but avoided as an antidepressant due to excessive sedation especially at doses needed to effectively target depression. The atypical antidepressants do not have as much data available regarding safety, but can be assumed to be similar to SSRIs and SNRIs due to common mechanism of action. Based on the sparse evidence available, risks associated with these medications are assumed to be similar to SSRIs (Newport et al., 2014; Schatzberg, Cole, & DeBattista, 2015).

Risks of Antidepressants

Neonatal Adaptation Syndrome

Neonatal adaptation syndrome (NAS) refers to observed signs of neonatal distress immediately post-delivery. NAS is theorized to result from withdrawal from intrauterine serotonin and is considered analogous to withdrawal syndromes observed in adults who abruptly stop antidepressants (Stewart & Vigod, 2014). Serotonin discontinuation syndrome in adults is believed to result from an abrupt change in baseline neuronal firing rate established through long-term adaptation to an antidepressant (Stewart & Vigod, 2014). As the brain attempts to re-establish a baseline firing rate, it overcompensates, leading to an imbalance in neurotransmitter balance and over-activity of other neurotransmitters, leading to anxiety, hyperactivity, insomnia, irritability, dizziness, nausea, vomiting, chills and myalgias (Stewart & Vigod, 2014). In neonates, it is unknown if NAS is caused by abrupt discontinuation, antidepressant side effects, antidepressant toxicity or a combination of these factors (Stewart & Vigod, 2014). Many observed symptoms are similar to those seen in excess serotonin syndromes. Common symptoms of NAS include agitation/restlessness, continuous crying/irritability, poor feeding, hypoglycemia, hypothermia, respiratory distress, altered muscle tone/hyperreflexia, jitteriness, shivering, tremors and seizure (Stewart & Vigod, 2014). In general, most NAS symptoms are transient/self-limited and can be safely managed with close monitoring for 48 hours post-delivery. Current guidelines advise *against* discontinuing antidepressants in the third trimester because risk of mood or anxiety disorder relapse post-delivery is high and discontinuation fails to prevent many NAS cases (COPE Guidelines, 2011; NICE Guidelines, 2014; Stewart & Vigod, 2014; Yonkers et al., 2012)

Persistent Pulmonary Hypertension of the Newborn (PPHN)

PPHN is a potentially fatal condition in which neonatal resistance to pulmonary blood flow fails to lower after birth. Baseline rates of PPHN are estimated to be roughly 2 per 1,000 births (Stowe, 2012). Individual antidepressant studies examining risk have been contradictory (Ray & Stowe, 2014). However, meta-analyses of available studies demonstrate an elevated risk of PPHN with antidepressants (COPE Guidelines, 2011; NICE Guidelines, 2014; Ray & Stowe, 2014; Yonkers et al., 2012). The rate of PPHN with antidepressants is estimated to be 3 per 1,000 (Ray & Stowe, 2014; Stowe, 2012).

Pharmacotherapy for Bipolar and Psychotic Disorders

Mood Stabilizers and Antiepileptic Drugs

There are estimates that 20% of patients receiving antidepressant medication for depression have bipolar disorder (Merrill et al., 2015). Bipolar disorder carries a high risk of premature mortality due to higher risk of suicide, as well as effects of accidents, substance abuse and general medical disorders

(Viguera et al., 2007). Similar to antidepressant treatment in pregnancy, a common clinical practice is to stop mood stabilizer treatment during pregnancy to avoid adverse fetal developmental effects (Viguera et al., 2007). Unfortunately, due to the nature of bipolar disorder, even with treatment, 37% of patients in the general population relapse into depression or mania within one year and 60% relapse within 2 years (Cohen et al., 2006). Although treatment interventions for bipolar disorder includes therapy and social intervention, the gold standard for bipolar disorder treatment requires medication. Because of the severity and complicated nature of acute bipolar disorder, we recommend that bipolar disorder is managed by psychiatrists, preferably treatment by perinatal specialists and potentially in an inpatient setting. It is not recommended primary care providers be managing acute mania. On the other hand, in stable bipolar disorder, at times, obstetricians and family medicine providers may be asked to continue maintenance treatment for bipolar disorder. We will focus on the most common medications used in the treatment of *maintenance* phase of bipolar disorders (COPE Guidelines, 2011; NICE Guidelines, 2014; Yonkers et al., 2004).

Mood Stabilizers: Lithium

Lithium is one of the oldest medications used in the treatment of bipolar disorder. The term "mood stabilizer" was applied to lithium when it was discovered that lithium could alleviate mania as well as be used in the maintenance phase for the prevention of both mania and depression (Schatzberg et al., 2015). Lithium has traditionally been the first-line treatment for bipolar disorder, especially for Bipolar I or mixed disorder. However, given the risk of birth defects, lithium is not recommended by NICE guidelines unless an antipsychotic has been ineffective (NICE Guidelines, 2014). If lithium is required, NICE guidelines recommend clinicians counsel the woman about the risk of fetal heart malformations when taken in the first trimester, discuss that lithium will be secreted in breast milk, and emphasize that lithium requires monitoring throughout pregnancy (NICE Guidelines, 2014).

LITHIUM'S EFFECTS ORGANOGENESIS AND INTRAUTERINE DEVELOPMENT

The most well-known risk of taking lithium during pregnancy is a cardiac defect of a heart valve called Epstein's anomaly (Bergink & Kushner, 2014; Yonkers et al., 2012). Epstein's anomaly is a downward displacement of the tricuspid valve into the right ventricle along with variable levels of the right ventricle being undersized (Yonkers et al., 2012). The risk of developing Epstein's anomaly is rare, in the general population approximately 1 in

20,000 (Robinson, 2012; Yonkers et al., 2004). When used in pregnancy, this risk increases to 1 in 1,000. Potential cardiac anomalies caused by lithium can normally be identified on prenatal screening with a high-resolution ultrasound and fetal echocardiography at 16–18 weeks gestation (Yonkers et al., 2004).

NICE guidelines recommend that women who need to continue lithium in pregnancy have their plasma lithium level checked every 4 weeks until the 36th week (NICE Guidelines, 2014). After 36 weeks, lithium levels should be ordered weekly (NICE Guidelines, 2014). Additional precautions include adjusting the lithium dose based on lithium levels, ensure the pregnant woman remains hydrated with adequate fluid balance, ensure the woman gives birth in a hospital and ensure the monitoring of fluid status and lithium levels during labor. Once a woman goes into labor, lithium should be discontinued (NICE Guidelines, 2014; Stowe, 2012) because dehydration can occur commonly in labor. Dehydration can thus lead to lithium toxicity in the mother and infant (Stowe, 2012)

Antiepileptic Drugs

Antiepileptic drugs are increasingly becoming more common in the treatment of bipolar disorder. One of the more common antiepileptic medications used in bipolar is valproate (Depakote). Valproate was approved for treatment of acute mania in 1994, and since this time has surpassed lithium in popularity (Schatzberg et al., 2015). While valproate can be very beneficial, it can be risky to use in females of childbearing age. The majority of pregnancies are unplanned, and individuals with bipolar disorder may be at even higher risk of unplanned pregnancy due to increased likelihood of engaging in impulsive behavior leading to lapses in judgment. By the time such a woman realizes she is pregnant, the fetus is already exposed (Stowe, 2012). Valproate carries a six-fold increase of risk of major birth defects as well as long-term deficits that have been linked to the development of autism, memory deficits and a decrease in global IQ (COPE Guidelines, 2011). Both the NICE guidelines and COPE guidelines recommend against the use of valproate in pregnancy given the risk of significant teratogenic effects (NICE Guidelines, 2014). The NICE guidelines take a step further to suggest that clinicians should not offer valproate for acute or long-term treatment of mental health disorders in women who are planning pregnancy, pregnant or considering breastfeeding (NICE Guidelines, 2014). In similar fashion, NICE guidelines recommend against the use of another antiepileptic drug called carbamazepine (commonly use in bipolar) during pregnancy given the risks outweigh potential benefits. If a woman is on either one of these medications for neurological purposes, a clinician should refer or, at least, consult a perinatal specialist (NICE Guidelines, 2014). The only antiseizure medicine that is recommended to consider in pregnancy is lamotrigine

(Lamictal). While Lamictal still carries risk of teratogenicity, it is much less that of either valproate or carbamazepine. Lamotrigine has a relatively favorable reproductive risk profile (Clark, Klein, Perel, Helsel, & Wisner, 2013) and is the preferred option for women of childbearing age for bipolar depression. Lamotrigine has less severe side effects and has incidence rates of birth defects less than 3% (COPE, 2011) and is more tolerable with less likelihood of causing weight gain. However, it also requires a slow titration scale wherein it can take 4–6 weeks to achieve a therapeutic dose (Schatzberg et al., 2015).

Antiepileptic Drug Effects Organogenesis and Intrauterine Development

Antiepileptic drugs negatively affect fetal growth and development to include 2–7 times an increased risk for hypospadias, cleft palate, polydactyly, craniosynostosis and 12- to 16-time likelihood of spina bifida (Robinson, 2012). Antiepileptic drugs are often associated with "anticonvulsant face," where infants exposed in utero have mid-face hypoplasia, short nose, upturned nostrils and long upper lip (Yonkers et al., 2004).

In summary, not all antiepileptic drugs carry the same risk. The general adage is the stronger the drug/more effective it is in treating acute mania and/or seizures, the greater the teratogenicity. Given the side effects, many experts recommend that if a woman is on medication when she becomes pregnant, valproate should be switched to another drug (Yonkers et al., 2004). One potential strategy to offset side effects of medication is to supplement with folate. Antiepileptic drugs' primary effect on the nervous system is depletion of folate (Yonkers et al., 2004). In response, the American Academy of Neurology has recommended 3–4mg/day of folic acid (Yonkers et al., 2004).

Atypical Antipsychotics

In the past, antipsychotic medication was typically limited to treatment of psychotic disorders. With the development of a second generation antipsychotic (SGA) these medications have been used in the treatment of multiple disorders (Schatzberg et al., 2015). SGAs have been included in guidelines for treatment of mania but have also been used for the treatment of treatment-resistant depression, refractory anxiety, sleep disorders, self-harming behaviors and trauma-related disorders (Galbally, Snellen, & Power, 2014). Antipsychotics have more rapid onset of actions, less neurological side effects of first-generation antipsychotics, and they are efficacious in treating the maintenance phase of bipolar disorder and bipolar depression (Schatzberg et al., 2015). SGAs include one of two agents approved for depression-combination of olanzapine (Zyprexa) and fluoxetine (Prozac) as a combo medication called Symbyax (Schatzberg et al., 2015). The other medication used to treat bipolar depression is quetiapine (Seroquel), and it may even be effective in monotherapy (Schatzberg et al., 2015). There is emerging literature about a third SGA called Lurasidone. However, given the newness of this medication at the time of this manuscript, we have not included it in discussion.

Antipsychotic Drug Effects Organogenesis and Intrauterine Development

SGAs are associated with increased weight gain, increased cholesterol predisposition to metabolic syndrome and neurological side effects called extrapyramidal symptoms (EPS). Potential risks of SGAs in pregnancy increased the risk of gestational diabetes and subsequently increase the likelihood of high birthweight (Galbally et al., 2014; NICE Guidelines, 2014). NICE guidelines emphasize that although there are not significant risks for SGAs, the limited data does not mean there is no risk, but simply no data to suggest harm (NICE Guidelines, 2014; Stowe, 2012). NICE guidelines recommend that women are taking SGA be monitored for excessive weight gain (NICE Guidelines, 2014).

In 2011, the U.S. Food and Drug Administration (FDA) issued a safety warning that expressed concerns about potential for antipsychotic use with the association of abnormal muscle movements or EPS in a newborn infant (Galbally et al., 2014). Symptoms of EPS in neonates include motor restlessness, tremor, hypertonicity, dystonia and Parkinsonism (Galbally et al., 2014). These symptoms are usually transient and brief. Long-term detrimental effects in limited studies have found an association between in utero exposure to SGAs and early delayed motor performance as well as delayed cognitive, social-emotional and adaptive behavior on the Bayley Scales of infant development (Galbally et al., 2014). When observed for longer periods, these delayed milestones appeared to disappear by 12 months (Galbally et al., 2014).

The Art of Psychopharmacology in Pregnancy

Prescribing Ethics

More than any other area of medicine, pharmacologic treatment of mental illness in pregnancy requires that providers prioritize patient autonomy and truthfulness/honesty over other values of medical ethics such as beneficence, non-maleficence and justice. Most treatment decisions that patients and clinicians will make have the potential to harm the mother, the fetus, or both (COPE Guidelines, 2011; NICE Guidelines, 2014). There is also a possibility that a woman's treatment decisions made may lead to the involuntary or voluntary termination of pregnancy. Clinicians must take care to give patients all the information required to make an informed choice. The decision to treat with medication or not must be the patient's, and clinicians need to avoid pushing their values/treatment preference onto the patient (NICE Guidelines, 2014). A clinician needs to understand the risk of medication on the fetus, while countering with the risk of untreated depression or mania on the mother and the mother–infant relationship.

Treatment Decision Making

It is the clinician's role to present some acceptable treatment options and then allow the patient to choose between them. A clinician should discuss the risk of treatment (with medication) versus the risk of no treatment. Mothers who elect not to continue medications should be counseled about likelihood of relapse and psychosocial treatment interventions (COPE Guidelines, 2011; NICE Guidelines, 2014). Clinicians should also discuss that discontinuing medications after discovering pregnancy does not negate risk, and birth defects may still occur (COPE Guidelines, 2011). Clinicians should emphasize that there is still clinical uncertainty regarding risk and discuss baseline likelihood of birth defects for mothers regardless of medication use or mental illness (COPE Guidelines, 2011; NICE Guidelines, 2014).

A mother must decide what risks she is willing to accept in various areas by identifying what symptoms are most important to target in treatment. She may choose to discontinue all medications if she prioritizes the health of her developing baby over her own. Alternatively, if a mother prioritizes her health (taking medication when necessary), it increases the risk to the fetus, but decreases the risk of harm due to untreated mental illness. When presented the risks and benefits of each of these options, mothers frequently make the best decision they can, usually based out of their morality and religious beliefs. All treatment options have a clear downside, and no choice is clearly superior to the others. Each choice will have potential consequences for the mother, to the developing fetus or both. Our advice would be to provide all available evidence and allow the patient to make the best decision she can based on her morality/beliefs. The decision to screen for birth defects can also raise moral dilemmas, as some women may elect to terminate the pregnancy if the fetus is found to have birth defects. A helpful, free, up-to-date resource for clinicians and patients looking for more information about particular treatments is the Women's Mental Health Clinic at Massachusetts General Hospital website (womensmentalhealth.org). See Table 8.1.

Table 8.1 Prescriber Decision Making

Stops taking medication	Ensure adequate social support Discuss risk associated with stopping medication Offer psychological intervention
Medication is started during pregnancy or postpartum period	Choose drug with lowest risk Use lowest *effective* dose Use single drug Recognize that the physiological changes in pregnancy may lead to needing to adjust medications in various trimesters
Severe mental illness stops medication	Discuss reasons for discontinuance Discuss possibility of restarting medication, switching and/or having psychological intervention

Informed Consent and Documentation

Although there is a baseline risk for birth defects in pregnancy, there is a strong bias toward attributing all bad outcomes to psychoactive medication rather than other causes. Treating pregnant women will always carry some risk, whether this be a risk of untreated mental illness or a likelihood of birth defects due to medication. Not treating a pregnant woman also conjures risk due to untreated mental illness, which then increases the risk of adverse events. Regardless of how good a clinician's working alliance is with a patient, some adverse events may result in lawsuits for accusations of wrongful death, wrongful life and medical malpractice. Should this occur, the medical record is the single most important piece of evidence that either side will introduce. A well-written series of notes is protective, and sparse notes lacking clinical rationale or informed consent makes judgment against the clinician more likely.

Medico-legally, the best notes convey clinical rationale and reflect that proper informed consent, monitoring and safety planning were performed. For most clinicians, the only change necessary is a more robust plan section in the standard clinical note. Documentation should address why a particular treatment was selected, what risks this treatment poses and how the clinician intends to both monitor for development of these risks and/or reduce the chances of the risk occurring (COPE Guidelines, 2011; NICE Guidelines, 2014).

> Background summary: "Patient reports stable euthymia since the last follow-up. She denies all symptoms of depression and mania. She reports having continued seeing her psychotherapist on a weekly basis which she finds helpful. Lithium remains effective and well-tolerated with no reported side effects. Lab work obtained from assessments was unremarkable, demonstrating a lithium level of 0.7 and adequate

hydration status. She denies new relational, occupational, familial, or financial stressors."

(Documentation of Mental Status Exam)

Patient recently learned she was pregnant and estimates being roughly 8 weeks. An in-depth of discussion reproductive issues associated with lithium took place.

In addition to risks discussed when lithium was initiated, we discussed potential teratogenicity (including 10–20x increase in relative risk of Ebstein's anomaly), the need for monthly monitoring of blood levels and possible dosage adjustments due to changes in fluid status, potential difficulties in delivery due to hypotonicity, and need to obtain regular blood levels in the newborn if she decided to breastfeed. We also discussed the need for routine fetal cardiac screening as the fetus has already been exposed to lithium for 8 weeks.

After discussion of potential risks, benefits, and alternative treatments, the patient elected to remain on lithium at its current dose. The decision to continue lithium was made due to nearly lethal suicide attempt made previous to starting lithium, previous treatment failures involving valproate, oxcarbazepine, lamotrigine, aripiprazole, and lurasidone, and the fetus having already been exposed to lithium for 8 weeks while organs were forming. Plan to increase the frequency of follow-up, clinical monitoring and laboratory testing to monthly and maintain regular contact with her psychotherapist. Due to her previous suicide attempt, she is considered a MODERATE risk for self-harm. The patient is considered LOW risk for harm to others. We reviewed her safety plan, and patient understands warning signs and symptoms which should prompt her to seek help, such as feeling isolated from supports, seeing herself as a burden to others, and persistent psychomotor slowing. She identified her husband Bill (555-555-5555) and her best friend Jane (555-555-5555) as trusted supports. She knows that she can also present to this office, her therapist, the nearest ER, or call the National Suicide Prevention Lifeline (1-800-273-8255). The patient's best contact number is 555-555-5555.

Severe Mental Illness and Safety

Postpartum psychosis is a psychiatric emergency. As discussed in Chapter 2, postpartum psychosis has a rapid onset and presents with bizarre delusions, mood swings, disorganized behaviors and significantly increases the risk of self-harm or harm to the infant (Sit, Rothchild, & Wisner, 2006). Postpartum psychosis requires emergency evaluation for medical causes and most always requires hospitalization (Sit et al., 2006). A woman who is acutely suicidal, homicidal or psychotic requires hospitalization (Lindahl, Pearson, & Colpe,

2005). Treatment then requires a differential diagnosis of underlying causes and educating the patient and family about the diagnosis. In bipolar and psychotic disorder, pharmacotherapy should be one of first treatments implemented (Sit et al., 2006) as well as acute stabilization, most often in the inpatient setting (Sit et al., 2006). Treatment of pregnant mothers in inpatient settings should be managed collaboratively by obstetricians and psychiatrists.

Hospitalization

Although hospitalization is one of the last modalities of treatment used, it is often viewed negatively. While postpartum psychosis necessitates admission, the majority of admissions are due to severe anxiety/depression. Many depressed mothers may already be struggling with bonding/relating to the infant, and fear that hospitalization will continue to separate them from their baby and further worsen the mother–infant bond. Fortunately, there is an option to stabilize the mother in an inpatient study, while also addressing the mother–infant bond. There are select hospitals throughout the United States that have a Psychiatric Mother Baby Unit (MBUs). MBUs allow joint admission of mothers with their infants (Christl, Reilly, Yin, & Austin, 2015). MBUs allow mothers to receive psychiatric care during the postpartum period and at the same time support the development of parenting skills and infant bonding and prevent the potential negative effects of a separation on a women's confidence in parenting and developing an attachment with an infant (Christl et al., 2015). MBUs started in Great Britain in 1958 and since this time have spread throughout various countries (Christl et al., 2015). In 2011, the first MBU opened in the United States at the University of North Carolina, Chapel Hill (Stampler, 2011). MBUs have a growing amount of research to identify positive outcomes/advantages to admission with the infant instead of standard psychiatric admission (Christl et al., 2015). For women admitted with unipolar depression and anxiety disorders, some MBUs have a symptom recovery rate of 73.3% (Christl et al., 2015).

After discharge from the inpatient setting, there are also mother–baby partial hospitalization programs that are less intensive or restrictive, but allow mother and infant to seek joint treatment. In a partial hospital setting, women typically attend for 6–8 hours a day, up to 5 days a week. Like MBUs, there are only a select number of mother–baby partial hospitalization programs in the United States. Table 8.2 will discuss the various current partial programs and inpatient programs within the United States.

ECT and TMS in Pregnancy/Postpartum

At times, pharmacotherapy/psychotherapy and social interventions are not sufficient to treat psychosis/severe depression or mania. In these cases, Electroconvulsive Therapy (ECT) may be an option (COPE Guidelines, 2011;

Table 8.2 Perinatal Partial Programs and Mother Baby Units

Program	*Type*	*Description*
UNC Perinatal Psychiatric Inpatient Unit Chapel Hill, NC	Inpatient and Day Treatment (also has outpatient program)	Psychiatric inpatient unit (secure unit) for psychiatric stabilization, but treatment includes medication management, supportive therapy, education, occupational therapy, recreation therapy and nutrition counseling, while assisting in care of newborn. Admission usually last 7–14 days
Brown/Women & Infants Providence, RI	Day Hospital	Opened February 2000 and has treated > 3,000 pregnant and postpartum patients
El Camino Hospital Maternal Outreach Mood Services (MOMs) Mountain View, CA	Outpatient treatment Day treatment program	Day program that includes individual, couples and group counseling —
San Diego Maternal Mental Health Program San Diego, CA	Outpatient treatment	Outpatient clinic created in 2007 to help women recover from anxiety, depression or emotional concerns during pregnancy or postpartum period
Huntington Memorial Hospital Maternal Wellness Program	Inpatient program	Inpatient 4-bed unit that is tailored to needs of women and their children, in particular mother–child bonding and attachment

Source: Adapted from Postpartum Support International website: http://www.postpartum.net/professionals/intensive-perinatal-psych-treatment-in-the-us/

NICE Guidelines, 2014). ECT can be used in either pregnancy or postpartum period (Jones, Chandra, Dazzan, & Howard, 2014). During pregnancy, ECT should be considered in pregnant women who are acutely suicidal, in stupor/catatonic or psychotic (Jones et al., 2014). ECT is also used in women with severe depression, women with severe mixed affective states, women with catatonia (NICE Guidelines, 2014). Women with postpartum psychosis respond very well to ECT (Sit et al., 2006). ECT is an option when patients have failed drug therapy, cannot wait for delayed onset of action of drugs, patients who require rapid treatment efficacy, or present with gross impairments in self-care/cognition and function. ECT can cause rapid improvement and is the treatment of choice in severe psychotic disorders or catatonia (Garcia, Flynn, Pierce, & Caudle, 2010). Additionally, although ECT does not require prolonged use of medications, the initial treatment needs to be performed in a hospital under anesthesia.

In addition to ECT, there is another somatic treatment modality available for treatment of severe depression called Transcranial Magnetic Stimulation

(TMS). TMS is rapidly becoming a popular treatment modality in pregnancy and postpartum to treat treatment-resistant depression and or psychosis/bipolar disorder as well as individuals unable to take medication. TMS uses briefly pulsed, powerful magnetic fields to induce an electrical current in the brain (Garcia et al., 2010). TMS can alter regional activity in the brain without causing diffuse effects that occur in ECT and transmit electrical impulses that travel along existing neurological pathways and stimulate one side of the brain then induce changes in the opposite side of the brain (Gershon, Dannon, & Grunhaus, 2003). TMS is also thought to alter neurotransmitter release from neurons and increase the release of dopamine (Gershon et al., 2003). Some of the theories behind the benefits of TMS are based on the premise that depressed patients have less blood flow and hypometabolism in left prefrontal cortex (Sayar et al., 2014). The two main types of TMS are divided by the frequency of electrical discharge; high frequency or low frequency. One type is called high-frequency rTMS and is applied to the left prefrontal cortex, while low-frequency rTMS is applied to right prefrontal cortex (Sayar et al., 2014). High-frequency TMS causes excitability in the brain and increases metabolism while low frequency does the opposite (Gershon et al., 2003).

Like ECT, TMS can be effective in treatment-refractory patients, or in patients who desire to avoid drug therapy. TMS is noninvasive, simple, safe with rapidly improving technology (Sayar et al., 2014). In 2008, the FDA approved TMS as an alternative form of treating treatment-resistant depression (Sayar et al., 2014). Response to TMS can occur in as little as 2–4 weeks, and this response can be sustained (Garcia et al., 2010). TMS is an outpatient treatment that does not require the use of anesthesia, and patients can return to work immediately post treatment (Garcia et al., 2010). In an open-labeled study on using repetitive TMS (rTMS) in women with postpartum depression, TMS treatment yielded a rapid, robust and durable response and that allowed mothers to remain medication free until they were no longer breastfeeding (Garcia et al., 2010). Another study about use of TMS during pregnancy also found that patients receiving rTMS responded rapidly in as little as 2–4 weeks (Sayar et al., 2014). This study also proposed that rTMS was a more favorable treatment option for a woman with severe depression (although not psychosis) than ECT due to significantly fewer side effects (Sayar et al., 2014).

Medication Summary

Management of medication in pregnancy involves accepting calculated risk(s) for the benefit of a pregnant patient and her unborn child. Perfect solutions are impossible, and treatment goals differ from usual practices in that symptoms are held at a manageable level rather than seeking complete remission. With all treatment decisions, informed consent and patient autonomy should be prioritized over other ethical principles as all options carry risk to the mother, the fetus, or both. Antidepressants are the medications most often managed in primary care level, while bipolar medications require a psychiatric specialist, preferably a perinatal psychiatrist if one is available. In general, SSRIs such as sertraline and fluoxetine are seen as the safest options for treatment. When utilized, medications should be used at the lowest effective dosage and for the shortest duration possible. Polypharmacy is heavily discouraged. Arrangements/contingencies for complications during delivery should be planned for at the outset of treatment.

Take Home Tips for Pharmacologic Treatment of Pregnant Patients

(COPE Guidelines, 2011; NICE Guidelines, 2014; Ray & Stowe, 2014).

Remember

a) **The primary goal when using psychoactive medications in pregnancy is the minimization of potential harm.** Ideal pharmacologic management involves the smallest number of medications at the lowest possible dose. Non-pharmacologic interventions, such as psychotherapy, should be utilized whenever possible to reduce or avoid medication use. Augmentation with additional psychoactive medications should be avoided whenever possible (COPE, 2011; NICE, 2014; Ray & Stowe, 2014).
b) **Sometimes, the best thing to do is nothing.** Mild symptoms or sudden worsening of symptoms does not always require a clinician to change the treatment plan. Avoid the tendency to intensify treatment when symptoms are otherwise tolerable. Remission is *not* the goal of treatment during pregnancy. To minimize fetal medication exposure, treatment goals should change to symptoms which are tolerable and pose no risk to safety.
c) **Follow-up and drug monitoring need to occur more frequently in pregnancy.** Bodily changes due to pregnancy can destabilize previously stable patients, and side effects/adverse events can occur quickly. Pregnancy should be seen as a risk factor for relapse of mental illness and suicide, *not* a protective factor. Involvement of at least one of the patient's supports in the treatment plan can be beneficial as well.
d) **When medications have been discontinued, try to maintain the period off of medications for as long as possible.** Rather than holding medications for predefined periods of time (e.g., the

first trimester), base the decision to restart medication on the patient's symptoms. Often, medication can be held for far longer than originally anticipated before symptoms reemerge. We have been surprised in some cases where we were able to hold medication throughout the entire pregnancy despite concerns due to a patient's previous psychiatric history. The decision to discontinue all medications is not made lightly and should not be discarded lightly once that course has started.

e) **Clinicians are not locked into treatment if something is not working or the patient has side effects.** It is better to be wrong and change then to stubbornly continue a treatment that is not working (assuming the patient has had an adequate trial of the medication).

f) **Clinicians are not an island, and one does not have to know everything.** It is fine (often preferable) to call a colleague for advice, defer making a medical decision until reference material is consulted, or call a specialist before making an important treatment decision. Patients are typically grateful when clinicians demonstrate this level of concern and self-awareness. Be sure to document consultation with other clinicians in the medical record as this is protective from a medico-legal standpoint. Documentation is essential when consultation leads to a change in treatment strategy.

g) **Always think two to three moves ahead.** Providers should have several treatment moves planned out, which then leads to optimal informed consent. Furthermore, planning ahead enables providers to becoming overwhelmed/paralyzed if a treatment does not work, or the patient develops significant side effects.

h) **Try to anticipate likely treatments by other providers.** Many women receive epidural anesthesia and opiates when they deliver vaginally. The cesarean section usually involves standard surgical sedation. Certain medications are preferred in gestational diabetes and gestational hypertension. Select psychoactive medications that do not have significant interactions with medications used in labor or delivery and try to choose psychoactive medications that have dual benefits such as also being effective for multiple conditions. Providers should also communicate and collaborate with other providers involved in a patient's care to obtain better outcomes and reduce the likelihood of polypharmacy dangerous drug–drug interactions.

i) **Do not be afraid to advise a patient to defer taking another clinician's medication or ask that the patient not start any new medications until it has been verified that no drug–drug interactions exist.** When patients have multiple clinicians across different specialties, the likelihood of polypharmacy and significant drug–drug interaction rises. Co-morbidities of particular concern when treating behavioral health conditions are chronic pain, migraines and hypertension, which can lead to the initiation of multiple antidepressants (particularly tricyclic antidepressants), initiation of multiple antiepileptics, initiation of medications that alter metabolism/clearance of other medications, and/or abrupt discontinuation of behavioral health medications. Medication reconciliation needs to be performed at every encounter. Consultation with the patient's other clinician is advised whenever this occurs so that all clinicians can provide uniform guidance to the patient. Worst case scenario in doing this is a clinician may be wrong and learn something.

j) **Run medication regimens of three or more medications through a drug–drug interaction checker, particularly regimens including tricyclic antidepressants, anti-epileptics or monoamine oxidase inhibitors.** There are free drug–drug interaction checkers that are found online. Common drug interactions include tricyclic antidepressants combined with other antidepressants—levels of both increase due to competition for the same CYP450 enzyme(s); lithium combined with diuretics (certain diuretics increase lithium levels by inhibiting renal clearance); topiramate combined with many antipsychotics (topiramate lowers blood levels of many antipsychotics through induction of a particular CYP450 enzyme); and valproate combined with lamotrigine (very potent inhibition of metabolism requiring special dosing). Medications with very long half-lives such as fluoxetine are more likely to interfere with other drugs compared to drugs with shorter half lives such as paroxetine and venlafaxine.

k) **ECT, psychotherapy and other non-pharmacologic treatment options can be utilized at any time.** Other treatment options exist beyond medication. Pharmacologic treatment does not always have to be intensified, particularly if doing so poses significant risks for the patient. Avoid the trap of thinking every symptom needs to be treated with medication(s).

l) **Counsel pregnant patients about illicit drugs, St. John's Wort and S-adenosylmethionine (SAMe).** In clinical practice, there are patients whom idealize substances not regulated by the FDA, whether such be supplements or illicit drugs. Among illicit drugs, this is most common with marijuana. Patients are also often ignorant of the fact that over the counter St. John's Wort and SAMe are unregulated antidepressants in the United States. St. John's Wort, in particular, has a large number of drug–drug interactions, and SAMe drug–drug interactions are possible. Teratogenicity data for St. John's Wort and SAMe are sparse and contradictory (Dugoua, Mills, Perri, & Koren, 2006; www.womensmentalhealth.org). Current safety data are far stronger for FDA-approved medications than for St. John's Wort or SAMe (Dugoua et al., 2006; www.womensmentalhealth.org).

Military Family and Pharmacological Treatment

Military families have access to most treatment modalities discussed in this chapter. Most of the medications discussed in this chapter are on the TRICARE formulary. Many larger military treatment facilities have ECT as well as TMS. The only limitation is availability of intensive outpatient treatment program or inpatient treatment in the military health system. It is becoming more frequent that military treatment facilities have to rely on civilian network facilities to provide this type of care. Given limitation or inpatient treatment/on-post outpatient intensive programs, the military does not have any specialized mother–baby programs. Consistent with guidelines, most military providers attempt psychosocial interventions initially in the treatment of perinatal mood and anxiety disorders. The next three chapters will discuss psychosocial interventions at various levels of primary care: obstetrics, pediatrics/family medicine, as well as behavioral health.

References

American Psychological Association. (2014). Briefing Series on the Role of Psychology in Health Care. Perinatal Depression. Washington, DC: Author.

Bergink, V., & Kushner, S. (2014). Lithium during pregnancy. *American Journal of Psychiatry, 171*(7), 712–715. PMID: 24980165. doi: 10.1176/appi.ajp.2014.14030409

BeyondBlue. (2011). Clinical Practice Guidelines (COPE): Depression and Related Disorders- Anxiety, Bipolar Disorder and Puerperal Psychosis-in the Perinatal Period- A Guidelines for Primary Care Health Professionals. Australian Government: National Health and Medical Research Counsel. Retrieved from www.beyondblue.org.au

Chaudron, L. (2013). Complex challenges in treating depression during pregnancy. *American Journal of Psychiatry, 170*(1), 12–20. doi: 10.1176/appi.ajp.2012.12040440.

Christl, B., Reilly, N., Yin, C., & Austin, M.-P. (2015). Clinical profile and outcomes of women admitted to a psychiatric mother-baby unit. *Archives of Women's Mental Health, 18*(6), 805–816. doi: 10.1007/s00737-014-0492-x.

Clark, C., Klein, A., Perel, J., Helsel, J., & Wisner, K. (2013). Lamotrigine dosing for pregnant patients with bipolar disorder. *American Journal of Psychiatry, 170*, 1240–1247.

Cohen, L., Alschuler, L., Harlow, B., Nonacs, R., Newport, J., Viguera, A., . . . Stowe, Z. (2006). Relapse of major depression during pregnancy in women who maintain or discontinue antidepressant treatment. *Journal of the American Medical Association, 295*(5), 499–507. Retrieved from https://www.ncbi.nlm.nih.gov/pubmed/16449615

Cohen, L., Wang, B., Nonacs, R., Viguera, A., Lemon, E., & Freeman, M. (2010). Treatment of mood disorders during pregnancy and postpartum. *Psychiatric Clinics North America, 33*, 273–293.

Deneke, Edward. (2015). Screening for depression in the primary care population. *Psychiatric Clinics of North America, 38*, 23–43.

Dugoua, J. J., Mills, E., Perri, D., & Koren, G. (Fall 2006). Safety and efficacy of St. John's wort (hypericum) during pregnancy and lactation. *Canadian Journal of Clinical Pharmacology., 13*(3), e268–e276. Retrieved from https://www.ncbi.nlm.nih.gov/pubmed/17085775

Galbally, M., Snellen, M., & Power, J. (2014). Antipsychotic drugs in pregnancy: A review of their maternal and fetal effects. *Therapeutic Advances in Drug Safety, 5*(2), 100–109.

Garcia, K., Flynn, P., Pierce, K., & Caudle, M. (2010). Repetitive transcranial magnetic stimulation treats postpartum depression. *Brain Stimulation, 3*, 36–41.

Gershon, A., Dannon, P., & Grunhaus, L. (2003). Transcranial magnetic stimulation in the treatment of depression. *American Journal of Psychiatry, 160*(5), 835–845. Retrieved from https://www.ncbi.nlm.nih.gov/pubmed/12727683.

Goodman, J. (2009). Women's attitudes, preferences, and perceived barriers to treatment for perinatal depression. *Birth, 36*(1), 60.

Grace, S., & Sansom, S. (2003). The effect of postpartum depression on the mother-infant relationship and child growth and development. In D. Stewart, E. Robertson, C. Dennis, S. Grace, & T. Wallington (Eds.), *Postpartum Depression: Literature Review of Risk Factors and Interventions*. University Health Network Women's Health Program. Retrieved from http://www.who.int/mental_health/prevention/suicide/lit_review_postpartum_depression.pdf

Higgins, J., Altman, D., Cotzsche, P., Juni, P., Moher, D., Oxman, A., . . . Sterne, J. (2011). The Cochrane Collaboration's tool for assessing risk of bias in randomized trials. *British Medical Journal, 343*, d5928.

Jones, I., Chandra, P., Dazzan, P., & Howard, L. (2014). Perinatal mental health 2: Bipolar disorder, affective psychosis, and schizophrenia in pregnancy and the post-partum period. *The Lancet, 384*(9956), 1789–1799. doi: 10.1016/S0140-6736(14)61278-2.

Leigh, H., Stewart, D., & Mallios, R. (2006). Mental health and psychiatry training in primary care residency programs. Part II: What skills and diagnoses are taught, how adequate, and what affects training directors' satisfaction? *General Hospital Psychiatry, 28*(3), 195–204.

Lindahl, V., Pearson, J. L., & Colpe, L. (2005). Prevalence of suicidality during pregnancy and the postpartum. *Archives of Women's Mental Health, 8*, 77–87.

McInnis, M., Riba, M., & Greden, J. (2014). Chapter 11: Depressive disorders. In R. Hales, S. Yudofsky, & L. Roberts (Eds.), *American Psychiatric Publishing Textbook of Psychiatry* (6th ed.) [E-Reader Version]. Arlington, VA: American Psychiatric Publishing, Inc. Retrieved from http://dx.doi.org/10.1176/appi.books.9781585625031.rh11

Merrill, L., Mittal, L., Nicoloro, J., Caiozzo, C., Maciejewski, P., & Miller, L. (2015). Screening for bipolar disorder during pregnancy. *Archives of Women's Mental Health, 18*, 579–583.

National Institute for Health and Care Excellence (NICE). (2014). Antenatal and postnatal mental health: Clinical Management and service guidance. *Clinical Guideline*, December 17, 2014. Retrieved from www.Nice.org.uk/guidance/cg192

Newport, J., Fernandez, B. A., Juric, S., & Stowe, Z. (2014). Chapter 64: Psychopharmacology during pregnancy and lactation. In A. Schatzberg & C. Nemeroff (Eds.), *The American Psychiatric Publishing Textbook of Psychopharmacology* (4th ed.). [E-Reader Version]. Arlington, VA: American Psychiatric Publishing, Inc. Retrieved from http://dx.doi.org/10.1176/appi.books.9781585623860.as64

Osborne, L., Hermann, A., Burt, V., Driscoll, K., Fitelson, E., Meltzer-Brody, S., . . . National Task Force on Women's Reproductive Mental Health (2015). Reproductive psychiatry: The gap between clinical need and education. *American Journal of Psychiatry, 172*(10), 946–948.

Ray, S., & Stowe, Z. (2014). The use of antidepressant medication in pregnancy. *Best Practice & Research Clinical Obstetrics and Gynaecology, 28*(1), 71–83.

Robinson, G. (Winter 2012). Psychopharmacology in pregnancy and postpartum. *FOCUS Psychiatry, 10*(1), 3–14.

Roy-Burne, P. (2014). *Risks of Antidepressants during Pregnancy*. UpToDate. Retrieved from www.uptodate.com

Sayar, G., Ozten, E., Tufan, E., Cerit, C., Kagan, G., Dilbaz, N., & Tarhan, N. (2014). Transcranial magnetic stimulation during pregnancy. *Archives of Women's Mental Health, 17*, 311–315.

Schatzberg, S., Cole, A., & DeBattista. (2015). Chapter 3: Antidepressants. In A. Schatzberg & C. DeBattista (Eds.), *Manual of Clinical Psychopharmacology* (8th ed.) [E-Reader Version]. Arlington, VA: American Psychiatric Publishing, Inc. Retrieved from http://dx.doi.org/10.1176/appi.books.9781615370047.AS03

Sit, D., Rothchild, A., & Wisner, K. (2006). A review of postpartum psychosis. *Journal of Women's Health, 15*(4), 352–368.

Stampler, L. (2011). First U.S. inpatient clinic for moms with Postpartum depression opens. *Huffington Post* [Online Version]. 8/19/2011. Retrieved from http://www.huffingtonpost.com/2011/08/19/americas-first-inpatient-postpartum-depression-unit_n_931179.html

Stewart, D., & Vigod, S. (2014). *Infants with Antenatal Exposure to Selective Serotonin Reuptake Inhibitors (SSRIs) and Serotonin-Norepinephrine Reuptake Inhibitors*. UpToDate. Retrieved from http://www.uptodate.com/contents/infants-with-antenatal-exposure-to-selective-serotonin-reuptake-inhibitors-ssris-and-serotonin-norepinephrine-reuptake-inhibitors-snris

Stowe, Z. (2012). Psychopharmacology during Pregnancy and Lactation. Lecture presented at the Oakstone Institute Psychiatry Board Review Course, March 15, 2012. Purchased as a set from www.CMEinfo.com; Oakstone Publishing, LLC. Viguera, A., Whitfield, T., Baldessarini, R., Newport, J., Stowe, Z., Reminick, A., . . . Cohen, L. (2007). Risk of recurrence in women with bipolar disorder during pregnancy: Prospective study of mood stabilizer discontinuation. *American Journal of Psychiatry, 164*(12), 1817–1824.

Yonkers, K., Wisner, K., Stewart, D., Oberlander, T., Dell, D., Stotland, N., . . . Lockwood, C. (2012). The management of depression during pregnancy: A report from the American Psychiatric Association and the American College of Obstetricians and Gynecologists. *FOCUS: The Journal of Lifelong Learning in Psychiatry, 10*(1), 78–89.

Yonkers, K., Wisner, K., Stowe, Z., Leibenluft, E., Cohen, L., Miller, L., . . . Altshuler, L. (2004). Management of bipolar disorder during pregnancy and the postpartum period. *American Journal of Psychiatry, 161*(4), 608–620. Retrieved from https://www.ncbi.nlm.nih.gov/pubmed/15056503

Chapter 9

Military Prenatal Intervention Models

Karen L. Weis and Kelly O. Elmore

Prenatal Assessment and Intervention

In the antenatal period, maternal psychological health has received increased attention because prenatal anxiety and stress are associated with higher rates of spontaneous abortion, preterm birth (Roy-Matton, Moutqui, Brown, Carrier, & Bell, 2011) and low infant birthweight (Rondo et al., 2003). Consequences of negative maternal mental health can have an enduring impact on both mother and infant, which has led to an increased emphasis on prenatal assessment of anxiety and depression with appropriate intervention. While the idea of providing assessment and intervention seems relatively clear-cut, it is hard to develop assessment tools and interventions that measure and then appropriately address all the components of prenatal anxiety, stress, and depressive symptoms.

Prenatal interventions commonly focus on the promotion of early prenatal care and improving health behaviors (Feinberg, Roettger, Jones, Paul, & Kan, 2015). There is less focus on non-pharmacologic means of decreasing maternal stress and depression and little consideration to cultural practices, pregnancy expectations and the ability to systematically deliver an intervention to larger populations. Clinical relevant assessments and interventions require multidimensional approaches based on sound theory that can be extrapolated for use with a variety of patient populations.

Prenatal Intervention for Military Populations

Military life, separations, and wartime deployments increase psychosocial stress and depression for family members (Lester et al., 2013). Perinatal mental health stressors in the military population place Active Duty and dependent females at an increased risk of pregnancy complications and poor birth and infant outcomes as a result of the pregnancy-associated anxiety, stress and depression.

Before military deployments, the numbers of pregnancies increase in both active duty members and wives of active duty military personnel (Rosa, 1996). The separation that comes with deployment exacerbates pregnancy-related stress and anxiety experienced by military women. Haas, Pazdernik, and Olsen (2005) reported that over half of the highest scores for stress in pregnancy were reported for women experiencing partner deployment. Weis, Lederman, Lilly, and Schaffer (2008) found that women with deployed partners had the greatest anxiety with accepting their pregnancies and identifying with being a mother during the first trimester of pregnancy. Higher levels of anxiety persisted long after their partners' return and this anxiety affected postpartum role satisfaction (Weis & Lederman, 2010). On the other hand, women's self-esteem increased if they were able to remain in contact with their partner during deployment (Weis & Ryan, 2012). In another sample, women had higher self-esteem and lower anxiety if they had community support, especially if this was an on-base (military) support element (Weis et al., 2008). Given the benefit of community support, the use of support groups within the military community can be very beneficial and have been suggested to be used as the foundation for interventions with military families (Black, 1993). These support groups are optimized if they are led by military spouses who have successively navigated military deployments and separations (Black, 1993).

In congruence with Black's recommendations, research on military families validates that most military prefer not to participate in formal services led by professionals, but instead prefer self-help or support groups that emphasize personal growth and family adaptability (Black, 1993). Black's (1993) recommendations were purely addressing military family separations, but these same approaches can be extrapolated to apply to military families during pregnancy. Antepartum support groups in military families are particularly beneficial during pregnancy, especially for young women new to the military lifestyle. Women new to military life may struggle with the dual challenges of adjusting to role and identity changes for both pregnancy and military lifestyle.

In studies on military families, the wives of junior enlisted members tend to struggle the most with separations (Black, 1993; Orthner & Rose, 2005), and most significant, the families of young enlisted have higher rates/likelihood of child abuse (Gumbs et al., 2013). Given the risk factors for the military population, prenatal intervention is crucial in military families. Such need is what precipitated the development of a program of psychosocial support for wives of military personnel during pregnancy. The Mentors Offering Maternal Support (M-O-M-S™) program was designed specifically for military women, led by military spouses and focused on targeting psychosocial anxiety and stress of pregnancy by increasing resilience and adaptability.

Mentors Offering Maternal Support (M-O-M-S™) Program

The development of the M-O-M-S™ program occurred through a methodical process in which the results of a descriptive study of 421 military wives and mothers (Lederman & Weis, 2009; Weis & Lederman, 2010; Weis et al., 2008) were used to build the program elements. In this descriptive study, pregnancy-specific prenatal anxiety was linked directly to low birthweight and gestational age at birth for a military population (Lederman & Weis, 2009). To address these elements, the components of the M-O-M-S™ program addressed the following: concerns related to acceptance of pregnancy, identification with the motherhood role, well-being of oneself and that of the unborn child, feelings of helpless and concerns related to preparation for labor. These elements of pregnancy-specific anxiety were incorporated directly into the intervention because they were predictive of low birthweight and early gestational age (Lederman & Weis, 2009). Other elements known to increase prenatal maternal anxiety were added to the intervention program. The additional elements included topics on the changing partner/husband dyad and the relationship between the pregnant woman and her mother as well as anticipated challenges due to the family of origin (Lederman & Weis, 2009). Important aspects of a pregnant woman's relationship with her mother included the availability of the maternal grandmother, reaction to the pregnancy, respect for autonomy, and a willingness to reminisce (Lederman & Weis, 2009). For military women, the geographical separations from loved ones may intensify prenatal anxiety, particularly if there are difficulties maintaining frequent and sustained contact with family members. Generally, partner support is the greatest contributor to overall maternal well-being during pregnancy (Brown, 1986). Therefore, it is important that the pregnant woman has availability to communicate with her husband or partner regarding pregnancy and childbirth (Lederman & Weis, 2009). The M-O-M-S™ program delves into issues associated with relationship cohesiveness and adaptability and preparation for the inclusion of a new member of the family. In addition to the pregnancy-specific elements of anxiety, knowledge regarding the availability of military and community resources (both military and civilian) is essential for family development and cohesiveness. The women are given information regarding valuable resources for themselves and their growing family.

M-O-M-S™ Program Design

The M-O-M-S™ program is designed in an eight-session format, with sessions lasting one and a half hours. Each session mirrors a chapter in the manual created for the M-O-M-S™ program. The topics highlighted during each session of the M-O-M-S™ are aligned with pregnancy-gestational transitions and prenatal maternal anxiety concerns relevant to that timeframe of pregnancy. The chapters of the manual align with specific elements of prenatal pregnancy-specific anxiety (Lederman & Weis, 2009). Additionally, the manual is designed for fill-in-the-blank questions that require some introspection. These issues may require discussions with one's mother or husband/partner. While piloting the program, the women in the study identified a desire to have additional material on multigravida issues and postpartum concerns. These elements were added to the manual and incorporated into the intervention support program, with no extra length added to M-O-M-S™. Program attendance is designed to start in the first trimester when prenatal maternal anxiety is high (Lederman & Weis, 2009) and women are anxious to obtain information (Deutsch, Ruble, Fleming, Brooks-Gunn, & Stangor, 1988). With eight sessions offered every-other-week, the program lasts through the second trimester and at the beginning of the third trimester when the mother begins to attend other classes or programs (birthing classes, breastfeeding classes, epidural classes, etc.) in preparation for the birth.

Program Mentors

A foundational element of the M-O-M-S™ program is the concept of mentors facilitating the intervention. Mentors are selected based on their experiences as military mothers and wives and the attitudes they have regarding their experiences, the military lifestyle and their roles as military wives and mothers. Importantly, active duty and non-active duty women are encouraged to be mentors. An optimistic attitude and positive self-esteem are hallmark character traits desired in the mentors. The mothers within the groups act as mentors as well. It is not uncommon for multigravida women to be part of the M-O-M-S™, and they provide guidance and perspective on mothering and growing as a family within the military community. A 3-day training program provides mentor facilitators with the information they need to understand the underlying theoretical foundations of the program, the concepts they must cover during each session, and the importance of keeping sessions targeted to the key dimensions for that week. In addition to each session's targeted topic, there is the underlying component of family adaptability/flexibility, resilience, and coping that is interwoven through all the sessions. The mentor's experiences, coping strategies and discussions about flexibility within the marriage and family are essential elements for every session.

Program Effectiveness

Over the course of 5 years, approximately 300 women from a large military community, with over 230,000 military beneficiaries (MARCOA, 2015) were randomized to either the M-O-M-S™ program in addition to their regular prenatal visits or regular prenatal care without the M-O-M-S™. Women were invited to participate in the study if they were (1) at least 18 years of age, (2) a pregnant wife of a military service member or an active duty pregnant woman, or (3) in the first trimester of pregnancy. Women were excluded from the study if they were going to have a change in duty location during the research, or if they were pregnant daughters of military service members. The objective of the M-O-M-S™ program is to decrease prenatal maternal anxiety and depression, increase coping, resilience, self-esteem and maternal-fetal attachment. Each of these outcome variables was operationalized and measured at three time points (Table 9.1), once in the first trimester before entry

Table 9.1 Overview of Study Variables

Variable	*Measurement*
Prenatal maternal stress and anxiety—prenatal adaptation	Lederman Prenatal Self-Evaluation Questionnaire Short Form (PSEQ-SF), 53 items (7 scales) Higher scores on a scale indicate greater prenatal psychosocial anxiety. Biochemical markers of stress in labor, and labor and postpartum outcomes were used to provide convergent and divergent construct validity; Cronbach's alpha coefficients for the original PSEQ long form range from α = 0.75 to 0.92 (Lederman, 1996; Lederman & Weis, 2009). Weis obtained similar coefficients in her military populations. The instrument was factored with a military population and all 7 scales remained distinct. The 7 scales measure Well-Being of Self and Baby (7 items), Acceptance of Pregnancy (9 items), Identification of the Motherhood Role (9 items), Preparation for Labor (7 items), Fear of Helplessness and Loss of Control (7 items), Relationship with Husband (8 items) and Relationship with Mother (8 items). Each scale contains both negatively and positively worded items. The scales measure the level of anxiety the woman is experiencing relative to the particular dimension. Alpha coefficients for this study ranged from α = 0.75 to 0.92
Maternal-fetal attachment	Maternal Antenatal Attachment Scale (MAAS), 19-item scale. The internal consistency for the scale is α = 0.82. Higher scores indicate higher maternal-fetal attachment. Factor analysis yielded two distinct dimensions: Quality of Attachment (10 items) and Frequency of Attachment (9 items). The "Quality" dimension assesses affective experiences such as closeness, tenderness, positive feelings about the fetus, a desire to know it and mental representations of the future baby. The "Frequency" dimension assesses the intensity of preoccupation with the fetus (time devoted to thinking about, talking to, and dreaming of the unborn baby). The scale focuses on thoughts and feelings regarding the baby, rather than the pregnancy or the maternal role, which differentiates it from the Maternal-Fetal Attachment Scale (Cranley, 1981). Alpha coefficients for this study ranged from α = 0.77 to 0.83.
Self-esteem	Rosenberg Self-Esteem Scale (RSE), 10-item scale measures the degree to which one values oneself. The possible range of scores is 10 to 40, with higher scores indicating higher self-acceptance. The Cronbach's alpha reliabilities range from 0.84 to 0.90. The construct validity of the instrument was demonstrated by examining its conformity to theoretical predictions (Rosenberg, 1979). The test-retest reliability was found to be r = 0.85. This instrument was used in the pilot MOMS project with good results. Alpha coefficients for this study ranged from α = 0.87 to 0.90

(*Continued*)

Table 9.1 (Continued)

Variable	*Measurement*
Coping (measure of resilience)	COPE, 60-item scale measures 13 conceptually distinct scales related to active coping, the process of taking active steps and planning, thinking about how to cope with stress (Carver, Scheier, & Weintraub, 1989). Test-retest scores over a 6-week interval reflect relatively stable scores (r = 0.46–.86; r = 0.42 – 0.89). Convergent-discriminant validity was determined with moderate correlations with other concepts relative to coping: optimism, control, self-esteem, hardiness, anxiety, social blunting and monitoring. The Cronbach's alpha coefficients for the COPE scales range from α = 0.65 – 0.92). The authors indicate that all or some of the scales may be used. For the purposes of this study, the directions to the respondent will clearly indicate that the questions pertain to their ability to "cope" with military demands and lifestyle. Alpha coefficients for this study ranged from α = 0.86 to 0.87
Prenatal depression	The Edinburgh Postnatal Depression Scale (EPDS) is a 10-item self-report scale validated for use during pregnancy and the postpartum period (Murray & Cox, 1990; Thorpe, 1993). Scores range from 0–30; higher scores are associated with higher depression. Similar to the recommendations of Appolonio and Fingerhut (2008), scores of 12 or greater were associated with prenatal depression. The EPDS was the one instrument scored immediately following completion as participants scoring 14 or greater were referred for further evaluation. The Cronbach's alpha has been established as 0.80. For a military sample of over 400 women prenatally, the Cronbach's alpha coefficient was α = 0.86 (Weis & Lederman, 2010). Alpha coefficients for this study ranged from α = 0.86 to 0.87

into the study, once in the second trimester, at approximately 20 weeks, and again in the third trimester at about 30 weeks gestation. The women attending the M-O-M-S™ program were given the questionnaire booklets at the time of consent to the study, at class 4 and class 8 (if it corresponded with week 28 or later of gestation). The women in the control group were met at their prenatal appointments (corresponding with the above gestational dates) by a member of the research team and given the booklet of questionnaires.

Preliminary Results

The results provided are for preliminary analysis of 201 participant's completed questionnaire booklets for all three trimesters. There were statistically significant differences between the treatment (100 women) and control groups (101 women) for maternal age (TX, $M = 27.5$, $SD = 4.98$; Control, $M = 29.6$, $SD = 5.53$, $p = 0.01$), whether they were active duty (AD) (TX, AD = 49; Control, AD = 11, $p = 0.01$), and the number of prior deliveries

(TX, zero deliveries = 54; Control, zero deliveries = 28, $p = 0.01$). Of note, almost half of the pregnancies in each group were unplanned (TX = 44%; Control = 36%), but only two of the pregnancies were unwanted. In comparing differences across pregnancy between the treatment and control groups for each of the outcome measures, statistically significant differences were found for pregnancy-specific anxiety relative to *Identification of the Motherhood Role* (Control: $\beta = -0.27, p = 0.13$; M-O-M-S: $\beta = -0.6, p = 0.02$) and *Preparation for Labor* (Control: $\beta = -0.9, p = 0.02$; M-O-M-S: $\beta = -2.04, p \leq 0.001$). A statistically significant decrease in depression across pregnancy was found for the women in the M-O-M-S™ group (Control: $\beta = 0.36, p = 0.58$; M-O-M-S: $\beta = -0.94, p = 0.007$). Of note, the scores for depression in the control group rose during pregnancy. The M-O-M-S™ group also had statistically significant increases in the scores for resilience, while the control groups scores decreased (Control: $\beta = -0.07$, $p = 0.68$; M-O-M-S: $\beta = 0.41, p = 0.05$).

Not reflected in the statistics for the outcome measures were the mothers' satisfaction with the program. The majority of the mothers in the program told their friends about the program. The friends wanted to join, but for the study, random assignment to the M-O-M-S™ was maintained. The women asked to speak to the investigator so that they could express their feelings regarding the effectiveness of the program as they felt the measures were not reflective of the overall benefits. The wives of active duty members indicated feeling heavy pressure to support their spouse in his career. This feeling of responsibility was felt to have the highest priority, coming above their needs and those of their family. They felt their spouses were so involved in work that they were hesitant to ask for any help with matters concerning home or the family. The active duty women indicated fears that their pregnancies would have negative ramifications on their careers. Some of the active duty participants indicated they were trying to keep their pregnancies secret for as long as they could to decrease the likelihood of any ramifications. All the women in the M-O-M-S™ program voiced a desire for ongoing programs like the M-O-M-S™ that enable open discussions in a supportive, therapeutic manner. Additionally, the women indicated that the M-O-M-S™ program provided an opportunity to ask all the questions they were unable to ask for their prenatal appointments because of time and availability of the provider or clinic staff. Being able to ask all their questions and receive answers from both the mentors and other mothers was beneficial.

Implications and Recommendations

There is a growing body of science related to the psychosocial stress of pregnancy and poor birth and infant outcomes (Charil, Laplante, Vaillancourt, & King, 2010; McDonald, Kingston, Bayrampour, Doan, & Tough,

2014). However, there is a lack of longitudinal studies, testing the effectiveness of prenatal assessment and intervention programs for decreasing the psychosocial stress of pregnancy and depression, particularly within a military population. The preliminary findings from this study provide some evidence to support the effectiveness of a prenatal mentored-support program for decreasing the psychosocial stress of pregnancy and depression. The statistically significant decreases in two pregnancy-specific measures of anxiety, *Identification of the Motherhood Role* and *Preparation for Labor*, were important, in that both of these measures were found to predict gestational age at birth (Lederman & Weis, 2009). Anxiety related to *Preparation for Labor* was also found to predict lower infant birthweight (Lederman & Weis, 2009). Identification with the motherhood role is an intellectual task in which the gravida may or may not want to be like her maternal role models. Lederman and Weis (2009) indicated that this type of prenatal psychosocial stress is best addressed through supportive, informational interventions. The findings from this study support that assertion. Additionally, military women have voiced a desire specifically for peer-support programs. The decrease in depression scores for the M-O-M-S™ participants is also a significant result in that decreases in prenatal depression have been linked directly to improved mother–infant attachment (Dubber, Reck, Muller, & Gawlik, 2015) and child behavioral development (Moehler et al., 2007). Several women in the study had been unsuccessful in combating their depression through psychotherapy and pharmacological measures. They all indicated great satisfaction with the M-O-M-S™ program, and they had significant decreases in their scores over the course of pregnancy and participation in the program. Field, Diego, Delgado, and Medina (2013) compared the results of a group-interpersonal psychotherapy program and a peer support program and found that both groups had statistically significant decreases in depression, anxiety and cortisol values. There was a greater reduction in the peer support group's cortisol values. However, none of the scores showed a statistically significant difference between groups. The authors do note that the results provide evidence of the positive nature of the two programs. Field's et al. (2007) indicated that some of their results were not sustained over pregnancy. The design of this study prevented us from determining whether the decreases in anxiety and depression and increased resilience were sustained. However, the goal of the program was to affect birth outcomes. Given the results of earlier studies, the intervention focused on first and second-trimester psychosocial stress and anxiety. It was anticipated that decreases in the psychosocial stress of pregnancy would impact birthweight and infant gestational ages. While these results are preliminary and do not include birth outcomes, the findings are promising in that psychosocial stress known to predict both low birthweights and infant gestational age were decreased.

Mothers in Transition Program at Camp Pendleton

Naval Hospital Camp Pendleton (NHCP) is the Military Treatment Facility for Marine Corps Base Camp Pendleton. Marine Corps Base Camp Pendleton is the largest Marine Corps training base on the West Coast. Naval Hospital Camp Pendleton cares for both Navy and Marine service members and their families, retirees, reservists, and members of the armed forces temporarily assigned for training at Camp Pendleton. NHCP is a training hospital for family medicine interns and residents. There are approximately 120–140 deliveries at NHCP per month. The majority of these newborns have their 2-week well-baby checkup and follow-up care in the pediatric and family medicine clinics. Well-baby checkups occur at 2, 4, 6 and 12 months of age. Naval Hospital Camp Pendleton operates similar to smaller community-based hospitals in that high-risk pregnancies are referred to Naval Medical Center San Diego or other larger community hospitals in the area.

In June 2007, the Department of the Navy issued OPNAV Instruction 6000.1C. These directions from the Chief of Naval Operations gave specific instructions concerning pregnancy and parenthood. This provides guidelines for medical and non-medical management of pregnant naval personnel (servicewomen). Section 206 outlines specific instructions concerning postpartum depression.

> Medical Department staff shall routinely assess and screen all pregnant servicewomen and new mothers for signs/symptoms of depression or a history of depression/psychosis during the following periods of care: new obstetric care visit, transfer obstetric care visit, last trimester of pregnancy, 6 weeks postpartum as well as each of the well-child care visits in the first 6 months of life at a minimum as per DoD/VA Uncomplicated Pregnancy Clinical Practice Guidelines and American College of Obstetricians and Gynecologists.

Instructions noted that scientifically proven tools, such as the Edinburgh Postnatal Depression Scale (EDPS) should be offered to women in the postpartum period as part of a screening program for postpartum depression. The screening program is administered as a part of a woman's routine medical care and as part of her child's well-baby exam scheduled at 2-, 4- and 6-month intervals.

NHCP implemented the Perinatal Screening Survey program in June 2007. The goal of the Perinatal Screening program at NHCP was to reduce the adverse impact of depression on mothers, infants, and families' health. The screening identifies mothers who need to be assessed for education and appropriate referrals for treatment based on scores determined by the Perinatal Screening Survey, which was adapted from

Edinburgh Postnatal Depression Scale. Medication, psychotherapy, and group support are all appropriate treatments for perinatal depression. Naval Hospital Camp Pendleton protocol requires the Edinburgh Postnatal Depression Scale (EPDS) adopted format as a screening tool. The Edinburgh is a self-report consisting of 10 questions that are scored from 0 to 3 points and asks the mother to answer the questions based on how she has felt during the past week. Treatment guidelines from the BC Reproductive Mental Health Program describe seven different screening instruments that can be used to screen depression in adults; of these instruments, EPDS is the recommended screening tool for the perinatal period and is one of the most frequent tools used worldwide (COPE Guidelines, 2011; Williams, 2014).

The Perinatal Screening Survey is considered a modified Edinburgh Postnatal Depression Scale due to the addition of question 11 about deployment status of spouse and wording for question 10. The original question 10 asks about thoughts of harming self and NHCP question 10 asks about thoughts of harming self or baby. The Perinatal Screening Survey is given at the first OB visit, last trimester of pregnancy 28–32 weeks, 6 weeks after delivery and at the baby's 2-, 4- and 6-month well-baby checkups. When the patient comes in for her appointments or her child's appointments, the front desk staff gives her the Perinatal Screening Survey and asks her to complete the questionnaire. It takes less than 5 minutes, and when returned to the front desk, the staff scores the questionnaire, and the original copy is placed in her or her baby's chart for the provider to review during the appointment. The Perinatal Screening Survey copy is collected, and the information is entered into the electronic medical health record.

Scores less than 11 are considered low risk and educational material or referral to case management is offered as needed. Scores of 12 and above are considered moderate/high risk and patients are referred to social work for additional screening and appropriate referrals: therapy, support groups and assistance with medication referrals. All social workers at Naval Hospitals are licensed clinical social workers. They are trained, independent practitioners and have the ability to assess patients, diagnose and provide mental health services.

The authors and original participants in the development of the EPDS note in *A guide to the Edinburgh Postnatal Depression Scale* that they originally recommended a cut-off of 9/10 to identify the early onset of depressive symptoms. That was later determined to be over-inclusive, so a cut-off of 12/13 is now recommended. Research shows that the EPDS has been found to be valid during pregnancy. The modified EPDS question (pound symbol) 10 addresses the issue of thoughts of harm self or baby and requires an immediate referral without regard to the total score if a patient scores anything but zero. NHCP added a question to the EPDS for its population. Question (pound symbol) 11 asks if the spouse is deployed, preparing to deploy, coming home from deployment or not applicable. There have been limited reports about postpartum depression screenings at the military treatment facility and fewer studies about depression and deployment.

Military perinatal screening studies lacked post survey research which could further support formal perinatal depression therapy and support groups (Spooner, Rastle, & Elmore, 2012). Subsequently, the three sought to publish research and strengthen available resources for patients diagnosed with peripartum depression.

The study was published October 2012 in the *Journal of Military Health* and was completed at Naval Hospital Camp Pendleton (Spooner, Rastle, & Elmore, 2012). It was a retrospective cohort study using EPDS. They used 14 as the cut-off for positive screenings. The EPDS was modified to include a question regarding the status of sponsor deployment: no deployment planned, preparing for deployment, deployed or returning from deployment. A total of 7,796 surveys were available for analysis. The rate of depression was found to be 6.9% for active duty women and 4.3% for dependent wives. The rate of high-risk depression scores was double in women whose spouse was deployed during the initial obstetric (8.6% compared with 4.3%, $P = 0.04$) and the 6-week postpartum visit (8% compared with 3.5%, $P = 0.02$) compared to women whose spouse had no deployment planned. They concluded that the prevalence of high-risk depression scores during the "peripartum" period for active duty women and dependent military wives was similar to that of the general population; however, deployment status was a unique and significant risk.

Before 2007, NHCP did not routinely utilize screening tools for depression or keep statistics on women with perinatal depression symptoms. Beginning in April 2008, the hospital began keeping an informal count of women assessed positively for depression and screened by staff. From April 2008 to April 2009, 443 screenings by two staff licensed clinical social workers and one nurse case manager was performed. These screenings represented both servicewomen and dependent wives. Some women were screened more than once during their pregnancy and following the birth of their child. Resources and appropriate referrals were provided

Before NHCP began administering the Perinatal Screening Survey, the social work department received very limited referrals to screening women for depression during pregnancy and postpartum. That has changed significantly with the Perinatal Screening Survey. The survey has served an important function in the overall health of the women and their families being treated at NHCP. The screening gave providers an opportunity to learn more about the emotional health of their patients. It allowed providers to identify women that might need additional support, education, referrals or medications. It also financially justified the need for a full-time case manager in perinatal departments and licensed social workers to remain in the organization to care for this patient population.

Another major undertaking that came about as a result of the Perinatal Screening Survey was the creation of a support group for women facing issues of depression and anxiety during pregnancy and postpartum. The hospital sponsors a semi-monthly Maternal Infant Support Team (MIST) meeting. The MIST group is composed of hospital personnel: RN/OB case manager, maternal–infant social worker, division officers for maternal-infant departments, RN lactation consultant, pediatric newborn screening RN and representatives programs located on base: New Parent Support Program Director, Armed Services YMCA program director; Navy Relief Visiting Nurse; Military Outreach Ministry representative; Women, Infant, and Children (WIC) representative; community Public Health visiting nurse; and invited community program representatives. At several MIST meetings, it was discussed the number of women being identified as the result of the screenings and how to best support their needs. The Moms in Transition support group was created. The creation of this therapeutic support group was a collaborative effort between hospital staff, Armed Services YMCA, New Parent Support Program, and Marine Corp Community Services childcare program. The Moms in Transition group became a reality in direct response to the needs uncovered by administering the Perinatal Screening Survey. It is a 10-week support group for our female patients that have been screened for symptoms of depression and been referred to case management or social work. The group provides education and social support. It gives the participants an opportunity to build a support network. The Moms in Transitions group have been well received. The support group is for pregnant women and those parenting a child under the age of 12 months. Not all women referred to the group have chosen to participate, and an alternative information class for patients and partners could meet some of their educational and social support needs.

Also as a result of the study, the Perinatal Survey Screening forms were updated to include additional information. The new survey indicates an individual's status: active duty, single active duty or dependent wife. The survey used in this study did not separate single, active duty from married active duty members. It is possible that the increased prevalence of depression in active duty members could reflect the additional challenges faced by single, active duty members. The new survey has a place for providers to note any actions taken: referral to social work/case management, a prescription for medications, referral to mental health or no action taken. The additional information allows identification of interventions utilized to address perinatal depression.

Due to the prevalence of positive screening scores for depression at first obstetrical visits, information on perinatal depression is included in the prenatal classes offered at the hospital and on base. This introduces the information to prospective parents and educates family members about this potentially disruptive disorder.

All pregnant active duty military members receive their medical care at NHCP treatment facility. Not all military dependent wives receive their obstetrical care at NHCP; some are referred out to community providers based on where they live and the ability to provide care for expected deliveries for any given month. Not all children born in the facility receive their follow-up care in our clinics; many are referred to community providers. At this point, women outside our treatment facility may not be adequately screened for depression during pregnancy or postpartum. It is not known what the depression rates are for these women. Anecdotally, we know patients are happy with the resource but to expand and better organize future support groups, more research is needed. That may change as grants are awarded for screening and education.

Recently, the MIST group was dissolved due to competing interests. The focus now is strictly on using military resources to provide support groups. Those include moms in transition, new parent support, nurse-family partnership, black infant health services, focus project, family forces, family advocacy and the department of behavioral and mental health.

At this time, the NHCP department of OB/GYN has a case manager within the clinic who is available for scheduled and urgent appointments. This position has been invaluable to patients and women's health providers because immediate access is essential for starting and continuing care. It is tough for military families, spouses, and active duty to carve out time for another appointment. They may have limitations with access to transportation, childcare options and conflicts with work schedules.

The presence of a clinic case manager also changed the culture of providers referring for health services. There is a subject matter expert who can assist with mental health resources and take the time needed to explain thoroughly the services and provide close follow-ups.

For those clinics that do not have this available, the departments of OB/GYN and Social Work provide education to the patients through prenatal registration, centering classes and word of mouth to both patients and other providers in the hospital clinics.

One resource used in this program is the New Parents Support Group that provides in-home visiting with families. This program can be accessed stateside and in assignments abroad like Guam. The New Parents support program has been utilized by patients of various backgrounds, including patients who are also providers in the medical field. When providers experience this program from a patient perspective, it can help them provide insight and a personal touch when working with families.

Summary

Pregnancy and childbirth is an emotionally charged event affecting all cross sections of a family: the mother, the father and the extended family. The mother's prenatal psychosocial health is gaining increased attention as connections are made between prenatal anxiety, stress and depression to pregnancy complications, poor birth outcomes, increased incidence of postpartum depression and poor mother–infant bonding. These issues are particularly pertinent topics within the military given the stress compounded by separations and deployments within the military family. This chapter has identified two separate interventions provided in different military services that have the potential to be used as a models in other military settings.

References

BeyondBlue. (2011). Clinical Practice Guidelines (COPE): Depression and Related Disorders—Anxiety, Bipolar Disorder and Puerperal Psychosis—in the Perinatal Period: A Guidelines for Primary care Health Professionals. Australian Government: National Health and Medical Research Counsel. Retrieved from www.beyondblue.org.au

Black, W. G., Jr. (1993). Military-induced family separation: A stress reduction intervention. *Social Work, 38*, 273–280.

Brown, M. A. (1986). Social support, stress and health: A comparison of expectant mothers, and fathers. *Nursing Research, 12*, 414–418.

Carver, C. S., Scheier, M. F., & Weintraub, J. K. (1989). Assessing coping strategies: A theoretically based approach. *Journal of Personality and Social Psychology, 56*, 267–283.

Charil, A., Laplante, D. P., Vaillancourt, C., & King, S. (2010). Prenatal stress and brain development. *Brain Research Reviews, 65*, 56–79. doi:10.1016/j.brainresrev.2010.06.002

Deutsch, F. M., Ruble, D. N., Fleming, A., Brooks-Gunn, J., & Stangor, C. (1988). Information-seeking and maternal self-definition during the transition to motherhood. *Journal of Personality and Social Psychology, 55*, 420–431.

Dubber, S., Reck, C., Muller, M., & Gawlik, S. (2015). Postpartum bonding: The role of perinatal depression, anxiety and maternal-fetal bonding during pregnancy. *Archives of Women's Mental Health, 18*, 187–195.

Feinberg, M. E., Roettger, M. E., Jones, D. E., Paul, I. M., & Kan, M. L. (2015). Effects of a psychosocial couple-based prevention program on adverse birth outcomes. *Maternal Child Health Journal, 19*, 102–111.

Field, T., Diego, M., Delgado, J., & Medina, L. (2013). Peer support and interpersonal psychotherapy groups experienced decreased prenatal depression, anxiety and cortisol. *Early Human Development, 89*, 621–614.

Gumbs, G. R., Keenan, H. T., Sevick, C. J., Conlin, A. M., Lloyd, D. W., Runyan, D. K., . . . Smith, T. C. (2013). Infant abusive head trauma in a military cohort. *Pediatrics, 132*, 668–676.

Haas, D. M., Pazdernik, L. A., & Olsen, C. H. (2005). A cross-sectional survey of the relationship between partner deployment and stress in pregnancy during wartime. *Women's Health Issues, 15*, 48–54.

Lederman, R. P., & Weis, K. L. (2009). *Psychosocial Adaptation to Pregnancy: Assessment of Seven Dimensions of Maternal Role Development* (3rd ed.). New York: Springer.

Lester, P., Stein, J. A., Saltzman, W., Woodward, K., MacDermid, S. W., Milburn, N., & Beardslee, W. (2013). Psychological health of military children: Longitudinal evaluation of a family-centered prevention program to enhance family resilience. *Military Medicine, 178*, 838–845.

MARCOA Publishing. (2015, June 16). My Base Guide—Joint Base San Antonio. Retrieved from http://www.mybaseguide.com/joint_bases/67-1372/joint_base_san_antonio_our_military

McDonald, S. W., Kingston, D., Bayrampour, H., Doan, S. M., & Tough, S. C. (2014). Cumulative psychosocial stress, coping resources, and preterm birth. *Archives of Women's Mental Health, 17*, 559–568. doi:10.1007/s00737-014-0436-5

Moehler, E., Kagan, J., Parzer, P., Brunner, R., Reck, C., Wiebel, A., . . . Resh, F. (2007). Childhood behavioral inhibition and maternal symptoms of depression. *Psychopathology, 40*, 446–452. doi:10.1159/000107429

Murray, D., & Cox, J. L. (1990). Screening for depression during pregnancy with the Edinburgh Depression Scale (EPDS). *Journal of Reproductive and Infant Psychology, 8*, 99–107.

Orthner, D. K., & Rose, R. (2005). Deployment separation adjustment among Army civilian spouses. SAF V Survey Report, University of North Carolina at Chapel Hill. Retrieved from http://www.armymwr.com

Rondo, P. H., Ferreira, R. F., Nogueira, F., Ribeiro, M. C., Lobert, H., & Artes, R. (2003). Maternal psychological stress and distress as predictors of low birth weight, pre-maturity and intrauterine growth retardation. *European Journal of Clinical Nutrition, 57*, 266–272.

Rosa, C. (1996). Impact of pregnancy and pregnancy complications during deployment: The role of pregnancy screening. *Women's Health Issues, 6*, 361–363.

Rosenberg, M. (1979). *Conceiving the Self.* New York: Basic Books.

Roy-Matton, N., Moutqui, J. M., Brown, C., Carrier, N., & Bell, L. (2011). The impact of perceived maternal stress and other psychosocial risk factors on pregnancy complications. *Canadian Journal of Obstetrics and Gynaecology, 33*, 344–352.

Shea, S. C. (1998). *Psychiatric interviewing: The art of understanding a practical guide for psychiatrists, psychologists, counselors, social workers, nurses, and other mental health professionals* (2nd ed.). Philadelphia, PA: Saunders.

Spooner, S., Rastle, M., & Elmore, K. (2012). Maternal depression screening during prenatal and postpartum care at a navy and marine corps military treatment facility. *Military Medicine, 177*(10), 1208–1211.

Thorpe, K. (1993). A study of the Edinburgh Postnatal Depression Scale for use with parent groups outside the postpartum period. *Journal of Reproductive and Infant Psychology, 11*, 119–125.

Weis, K., & Lederman, R. (2010). Prenatal spousal military deployment and maternal prenatal adaptation as predictors of postpartum maternal-infant attachment. *SOJNR: Southern Online Journal of Nursing Research, 10*(3), http://snrs.org/publications/SOJNR_articles2/Vol10Num03Main.htm

Weis, K. L., Lederman, R. P., Lilly, A. E., & Schaffer, J. (2008). The relationship of military imposed marital separations on maternal acceptance of pregnancy. *Research in Nursing & Health, 31*, 196–207.

Weis, K. L., & Ryan, T. W. (2012). Mentors offering maternal support: A support intervention for military mothers. *Journal of Obstetric, Gynecologic & Neonatal Nursing, 41*, 303–313.

Williams, J. (2014). Best practice guidelines for mental health disorders in the perinatal period. *BC Mental Health.* Retrieved from http://www.perinatalservicesbc.ca/health-professionals/guidelines-standards/maternal (Accessed on 24 January, 2016).

Chapter 10

Military Perinatal Intervention Models in Pediatrics and Family Medicine

Kellie Haworth, Eric M. Flake, Michael M. Dickman, and Melinda A. Thiam

Pediatric and Family Medicine Intervention Overview

As we strive to better identify families affected by postpartum mental illness, it is well recognized that pediatricians and family medicine providers in the primary care medical home plays a significant role. The interaction and trust parents establish with their child's health care providers as they obtain routine infant care provides many opportunities for detection of parents struggling with depression or other stressors. Traditionally physicians are trained to focus primarily on their patient. For pediatricians, it has long been apparent that addressing family wellness is vital to the overall wellness of their patient, the child. For more than two decades, medical systems have evolved toward more comprehensive patient-centered medical homes. Those systems that care for children, such as pediatrics, have introduced the concept of a family-centered medical home recognizing that all individuals in the exam room, including parents and siblings need to be considered for optimal child wellness.

Why Pediatricians?

It is likely that pediatric providers will interact with mothers more often than any other health care professional will during the first year postpartum (Lofrumento, 2008). Babies under 1 year account for 74% of pediatric primary care visits with more than 25.6 million visit annually (Talmi, Stafford, & Buchholz, 2009). Obstetricians traditionally schedule 1–2 postpartum visits, after which mothers are referred back to their primary care provider who may not consider her role as new mother (Liberto, 2012). In contrast, pediatricians and family medicine providers have regular and consistent interaction with new mothers during several routine well-child checks that should occur throughout an infant's first year of life (Fleming, 1996; Lofrumento, 2008; Talmi et al., 2009). During these visits, pediatricians evaluate the infant's overall growth and development including whether the infant is reaching age-appropriate physical and intellectual developmental milestones as well as the infant's social-emotional development (Earls, 2010). As the mother–infant interaction is critical for the healthy social-emotional development of the infant, pediatricians may be first to notice maternal attachment problems when the infant demonstrates delay in social or emotional development. Pediatricians have opportunities at both preventive well-child visits as well as visits for acute illness to identify concerns likely to occur within the first year of life (Lofrumento, 2008). Often, recognizing these concerns can allow for early intervention and referral to a new parent support program and prevent later need for additional intensive inventions.

Why Military Pediatricians?

Pediatricians who serve U.S. military families are responsible for caring for children of current or retired service members. As discussed in prior chapters, there are unique stressors experienced by the military family that can affect the health and well-being of infants, children and adolescents. Military pediatricians, many whom have deployed themselves, have already been at the forefront of identifying how deployment affects children and families. Military families having unique lifestyles and cultural considerations often gravitate to medical providers whom share similar experiences. Families can expect both civilian and military pediatricians working within the military health system to be well versed in collaborative community efforts for child wellness as they provide a unified approach to promoting child resiliency. Pediatricians serving this unique population are subject matter experts regarding military childhood stress.

Pediatricians in the military health system are an indispensable asset in the critical mission of promoting resilient military families. These physicians weekly will have 100 face-to-face office visits, and 200 telephone contacts with military families with over 1,000 children empaneled to them for care. Additionally, they are directly responsible for the medical care and documentation of any special needs child in the Exceptional Family Member Program (EFMP). As pediatricians screen for signs of distress, they will provide direct family support and refer those in need of additional resources. Finally, military pediatricians can assist in a "warm hand-off" to base and community partners.

Family Medicine

Family medicine providers are the "ideal" providers to become involved with perinatal mental health. Known as "womb-to-tomb" medicine, family medicine providers can provide obstetric care as discussed in the prior chapter, provide care for infant as well, and provide care for the mother. Family practice providers are also skilled at the collaborative care and adept at working with other specialists in primary care such as obstetrics and gynecology, pediatrics and behavioral health.

Obstetrical inventions discussed earlier identified how women are screened at the primary obstetric visit, weeks 28, 36 and postpartum follow-up. Family medicine providers frequently screen for depression in adult populations with a two question depression screening scale called PHQ-2. Positive answers on the PHQ-2 trigger further screening for the potential disorder. Given that individuals or their family members with behavioral health issues often present to their primary care physician on an increased frequency compared to rest of the population, they have more opportunities to uncover a "positive" screening. Also, by establishing the rapport with individuals on a longitudinal basis, it may be easier to delve into chronic underlying issues. Family medicine providers are poised to provide comprehensive care of all members of the family that has been termed a "holistic family approach" because family medicine views the disease process in how it affects the family system, and how disease can affect different members of the family.

Military family medicine providers have unique advantage that they are able to understand the specific challenges associated with being in a military environment, whether this is related to combat or military life in general. Furthermore, family medicine provides an avenue of treatment for behavioral health care in the primary care setting. Behavioral health in a specialty setting has traditionally been viewed as stigmatizing due to the fear of how the behavioral health diagnosis will affect one's military career. Because family medicine providers provide treatment for the infant/child, active duty service member and his or her family, family medicine providers often have a unique opportunity to screen for behavioral health disorders and provide early intervention before it becomes a significant problem. Family medicine providers are skilled in educating patients and can use their rapport/alliance with the patient and family members to screen for mood/anxiety disorder, and identify potential internal/external barriers to care

From Screening to Assessment

Screening Recommendations

The American Academy of Pediatrics (AAP) Bright Futures Guidelines (2011) recognize the negative effect of untreated perinatal mood and anxiety disorders on the health of children. These recommendations encourage pediatricians to screen for caregiver depression at the prenatal visit, the newborn visit at 1 week of life and the well-child visits at, 1 month and 2 months of life (Earls et al., 2010; Fleming, 1996). Several depression scales and screens are available to health care providers that can assist in detecting red flags for parental stress and well-being. Feasibility studies have shown that new mothers can complete these screening scales while they are in the waiting room for a visit with the pediatrician of a family physician. The most popular, easiest, and most efficient of these screens is the Edinburgh Postnatal Depression Scale (EPDS). An alternate less specific questionnaire is the Parenting Stress Index–short form or the Perceived Stress Scale (Lofrumento, 2008).

Barriers to Screening

The AAP's Task Force on the Family stressed that pediatricians should have a family-oriented approach to improving family outcomes (Lofrumento, 2008). Despite the AAP's recommendation to screen for the presence of maternal perinatal mood disorders, many pediatricians remain unwilling to complete this important task. In a national survey of pediatricians, 57% felt they were responsible for identifying mothers who are depressed in the postpartum period, yet only 32% expressed confidence in their ability to diagnose perinatal mood and anxiety disorders (Lofrumento, 2008). Although the mother is technically not the patient of the pediatrician, maternal mental health screening should be approached similarly to other pertinent family screens, such as parental tobacco use, gun safety or other behaviors that put the infant at risk. On the other hand, some pediatric physicians do not perform screening for signs of psychiatric comorbidity but rely on their clinical observation skills. However, studies have shown that even well-trained pediatricians recognize only an approximate 25% of mothers with depressive symptoms and that higher detection rates are achieved with the use of validated screening tools (Lofrumento, 2008).

Other barriers to screening family members for psychosocial distress voiced by pediatricians include reimbursement and coding issues, confusion about appropriate charting, limitations of their scope of practice and time constraints during primary care visits. However, it is imperative to find solutions to these barriers, as unrecognized, and untreated maternal mental health issues are correlated with increased health care visits and poorer outcomes for their children. Additionally, untreated maternal mental illness has been shown to be accompanied by a significant increase in risk for infant abuse and neglect (Earls, et al., 2010). (see Table 10.1).

Observing the Infant and Mother–Infant Interaction

Although pediatricians' primary responsibility is for the pediatric patient, it is also critical that pediatricians consider the health of a mother. Pediatricians are uniquely qualified to evaluate infant development and mental health, through observation and examination of the infant's physical wellness and behavior.

In the process of evaluating infant behavior, a pediatrician is also trained to observe the quality of the mother's interaction with her infant and assess the availability of the mother as she relates to her infant. How a new

Table 10.1 Keys for Perinatal Mental Health Screening in Pediatrics

Screening Key Points
The key screening times: 2 weeks, 2 months and 4 months and 12 months. Symptoms usually appear 2–6 week postpartum and peek at 3 months*
The 4th month visit is very important, as unless baby has had severe colic, feeding difficulties or medical problem, most mothers begin to appear less exhausted, less anxious and even a bit more confident in their new role
Use of screening tools in pediatric office or during well-child visits identified 11%–13% of mothers who would not have been identified with clinical observation alone
By universally screening all mothers during the first year of life, identification of at-risk mothers improved from 1.6% to 8.5%.

* Permission to reprint information from Susan Dowd Stone

Table 10.2 Mother–Infant Interaction Types (Boukydis, 2012)

Interested and curious	Appropriately concerned and able to communicate and exchange observations and thoughts about their baby
Anxious and visibly worried	May want a lot of medical information, information about infant temperament/development hard to hear, distracted by events occurring in the room
Quiet and hard to read	Internally focused, less attention for interviewing, possibly tired and sad

* Adapted from Boukydis, Z. (2012). *Collaborative Consultation with Parents and Infants in the Perinatal Period.* Budapest, Hungary: Paul Brooks Publishing.

mother interacts through verbal and nonverbal behavior can demonstrate a reassuring attachment or red flags that require action. (Boukydis, 2012). See Table 10.2.

Observing the Mother

Mothers whom are struggling with depression or anxiety are often quiet and hard to read (Boukydis, 2012). Studies on the consequences of maternal depression to infant caretaking reveal that the presence of maternal depression/anxiety has a negative impact on preventive care practices, including the use of a car seat or attending well-child visits (Lofrumento, 2008).

Inquiring Further: Keys to Addressing Maternal Concerns

As potentially the first health care provider to identify a mother suffering from postpartum mental illness, providers must keep in mind both the importance and the delicacy of the situation. Pediatricians should be aware that when sincerely asking a mother "How are you feeling?," the responsive mood and verbal communication should match. When stated mood and nonverbal postures are not consistent, the implication is that the person responding is reluctant to disclose some particular information (Lofrumento, 2008). Some mothers may demonstrate a loss of eye contact, looking away, fidgeting with hands—some form of activity intended to divert attention away from the question in hand (Shea, 1998). These behaviors typically occur when a mother is experiencing internal turmoil from not wanting to lie, but also not wanting to disclose negative information.

Individuals with depression/suicidal ideations or whom are emotionally struggling often try to maintain a strong demeanor. If they believe they are portrayed otherwise, moms may psychologically label themselves as "weak" and assume the provider will judge them negatively. Identifying and labeling the clinical concern may pave the way for an open and honest discussion (Shea, 1998).

Recommendations of what pediatric providers should not say to mothers struggling in the postpartum period are mentioned in Table 10.3, while Table 10.4 provides constructive alternative statements.

Table 10.3 Keys on What Not to Say to Mothers Struggling in Postpartum Period

What NOT to say	*Explanation*
"This is a normal reaction all new mothers have."	Postpartum mood disorders are not normal and not all mothers experience them. Though "baby blues" is commonly experienced, this does not meet criteria to qualify for clinical symptoms that would impair normal functioning or require intervention, whereas postpartum mood disorders do.
"Don't worry about . . ."	Especially if a mother is experiencing symptoms related to anxiety or OCD, it is almost impossible for her not to worry. This statement discredits her symptoms and does not offer her the necessary validation that she is in fact experiencing symptoms which are stressful to her.
"A healthy baby is worth . . ." OR "You have so much to be happy about . . ."	Whatever a mother is experiencing, telling her that her child is worth it is not the correct approach. This author has encountered some situations where a mother did not in fact feel that the child was worth her symptoms, adding guilt to her resentment, which she ultimately perceived to validate her lack of emotional connection. Just as a provider would not tell a woman that her baby was worth the rape she experienced when she conceived, so they also should not express to her that her traumatic emotions and mental illness are worth it.
"You would never really . . ."	Do not dismiss a woman confiding that she is scared she may act upon an impulse or notion to hurt herself or others. Though in most cases (except in severe depression or psychosis) she will not harm herself or others, until she is evaluated, one cannot be certain. To ignore potential harm is not only unethical, but also illegal.
"Join a 'new moms' group."	Many mothers experiencing postpartum mood disorders feel as though they do not fit in with their "perky mom" counterparts. Often going to such social groups results in her feeling more abnormal and isolated.

What to Do With an Abnormal Screen

When routine screening identifies a mother at risk for a perinatal mood disorder, the pediatric provider is expected to first ensure the safety of the infant, the mother, and any members of the household. Though not expected to personally medically treat an affected mother, the pediatrician should be capable of providing reassurance and education. Referral to an Early Intervention Program for concerns regarding mother–infant attached is justified. The provider should supply a list of print and online resoures and be prepared to offer a referral to available local mental health professionals, support groups, or other therapeutic agencies. An immediate and emergent referral is warranted if the mother shows severe impairment, has comorbid substance abuse, exhibits signs of psychosis, displays behavior indicative of possible harm to herself or the child, or conveys suicidal or homicidal ideations. Frequent follow-up office visits are highly recommended.

Table 10.4 Key of What to Say to Mothers Struggling in Postpartum Period

What TO say	*Explanation*
"You are not alone."	Although prevalent, postpartum mood disorders are too often ignored or dismissed as cliché, with stigma surrounding even the discussion of them. Many mothers therefore feel isolated and alone in their battle.
"You are not to blame."	Mothers experiencing postpartum mood disorders very often have an overwhelming sense of guilt. They need to hear that this is not something they caused or could have prevented, and is not something they can control.
	Mothers sometimes need to hear that they have permission to seek help, that their mood disorder is treatable, and that their illness is temporary. Though they may not see the light at the end of the tunnel, to hear that it is there often will provide a hope they may not have had.
"With help, you will be well."	Mothers sometimes need to hear that they have permission to seek help, that their mood disorder is treatable, and that their illness is temporary. Though they may not see the light at the end of the tunnel, to hear that it is there often will provide a hope they may not have had.
"You are not crazy."	For most postpartum mood disorders, mothers experience a feeling of lack of control, stating that they feel as if they may be "crazy." Validation that they have an illness, and that it is not reflection of them as person or a mother can be relieving of substantial anxiety. For mothers experiencing postpartum OCD, informing that intrusive thoughts are different from psychosis is important.

A Real Life Example: Screening in a Military Pediatric Clinic

Pediatric and Obstetric Primary Care Screening at Fort Knox

Dr. Kellie Haworth conducted a Department of Pediatrics quality improvement project, partnered with the Department of Obstetrics and Gynecology while serving as an active duty military pediatrician at Ireland Army Community Hospital (IACH) in Fort Knox, Kentucky. The project involved the implementation of postpartum mood disorder screening using the Edinburgh Postnatal Depression Scale (EPDS) for all women (both active duty and dependent) encountered in the Pediatric Clinic during well-child visits throughout the first year postpartum and the first postpartum visit in the Obstetrics Clinic. The goal of this combined project was to initiate early detection and intervention. The Obstetric clinic screened during the routine postpartum check, which usually occurred between 6 and 8 weeks after delivery. In contrast, the Pediatric Clinic administered screens during the newborn visit, the 2-week, 2-month, 4-month, 6-month, and the 9-month well-child visits as outlined in Figure 10.1. A screen was considered positive

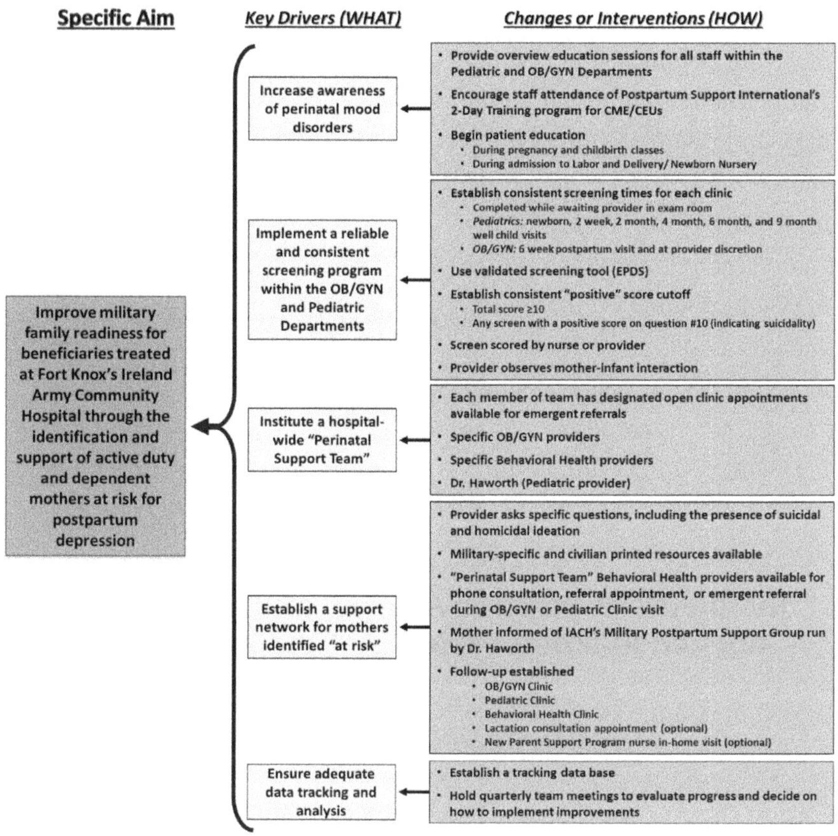

Figure 10.1 Process Diagram of IACH Screening Process in Pediatrics

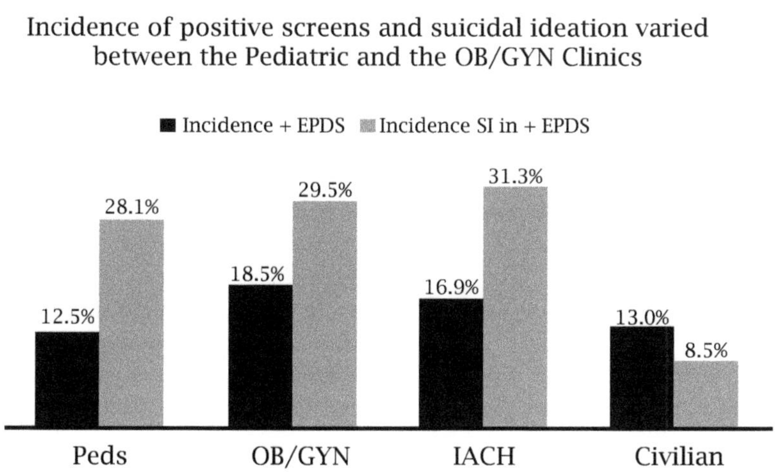

Figure 10.2 Chart on EDPS Incidence Between Obstetrics and Pediatric Clinics

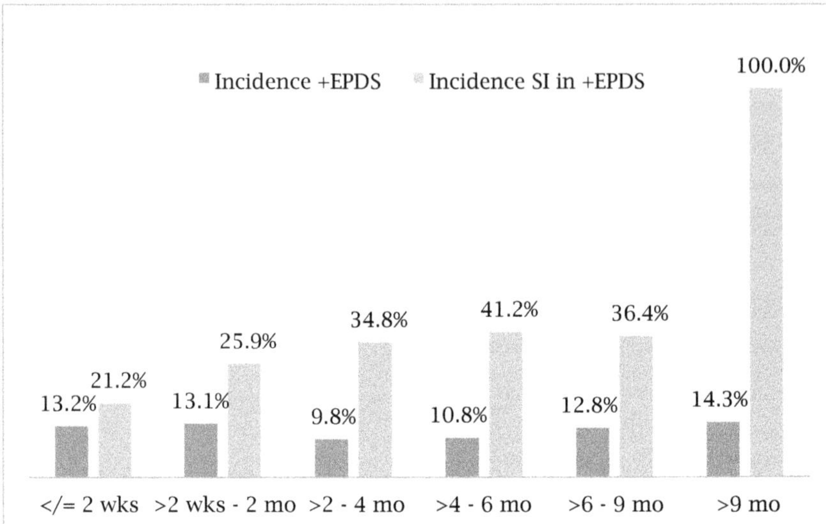

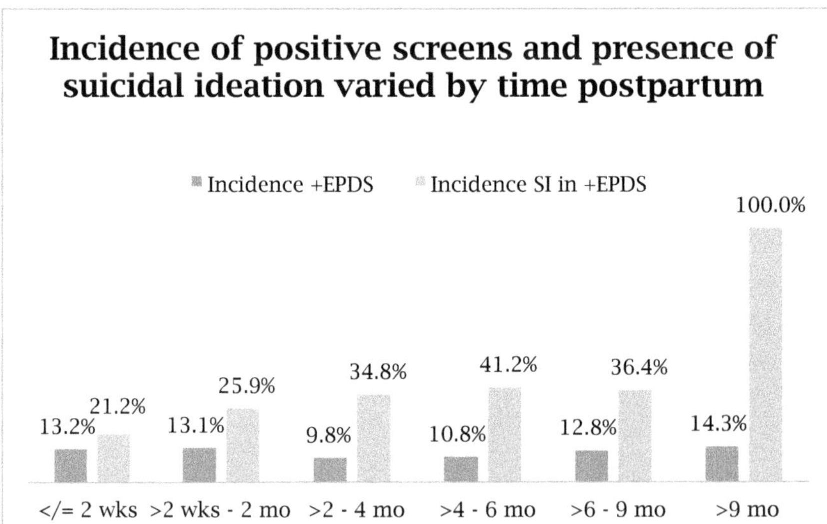

Figure 10.3 Incidence of Positive EPDS Screens at IACH

if the total score was 10 or greater, or if there was a positive response to question 10 (indicating the presence of suicidal ideation). A total of 1,877 EPDS screenings representing 1,043 women were obtained over an 18-month period. These figures are illustrated in Figures 10.2 and 10.3.

Pediatricians at Ireland Army Community Hospital addressed every positive screen with the mothers as they were encountered. The Pediatrics Clinics sent a nurse for specific training in perinatal mental health and utilized this resource to offer patients education, handouts, and a resource list. This nurse would also discuss the local support group (facilitated by Dr. Haworth), refer to the New Parent Support Program (which oftentimes provides in-home visits) and follow up via telephone. For mothers identified as high risk, the trained nurse would contact her obstetrician and/or the mental health clinic. IACH was fortunate to have the resources to develop a hospital perinatal mood disorders screening team that had established collaboration with two Psychiatric Nurse Practitioners and two Army enlisted mental health technicians from the behavioral health/social work department. If a mother required therapy, the trained pediatric nurse would assist her in making the appointment with specifically identified providers who specialized in perinatal mental health disorders. One note of importance: pediatricians were responsible for administering the screening, but they were not for diagnosing and treating. The beauty of collaborative care allowed pediatricians to screen, while also allowing a warm hand-off between the pediatricians and behavioral heath providers.

Integrated Treatment Team Models for Primary Care

Behavioral Health Integration into Primary Care (PCBH)

The Patient Center Medical Home-Behavioral Health (PCMH-BH) is a blending of two models of integrated behavioral health: the Primary Care Behavioral Health (PCBH) and prior Army model called Re-engineering Systems of Primary Care Treatment in the Military (RESPECT-Mil) (MEDCOM/OTSG, IBHC manual, 2014).

In the PCBH model, behavioral health providers called Internal Behavioral Health Consultants (IBHC) are integrated members who are part of the medical home. Despite being credentialed as behavioral health providers, they do not provide specialty behavior health, but instead provide expertise in health psychology and behavioral change. They can also offer brief, short term, solution focused treatment as little as a 30-minute consultation (MEDCOM/OTSG, IBHC manual, 2014). By being integrated into a primary medical home treatment team, IBHCs can provide a vital service to both patients and primary care providers by assisting with identifying and implementing effective and comprehensive health care plan (MEDCOM/OTSG, 2014). By being present in the clinic, IBHCs offer consultation to primary care providers and can ease the discomfort primary care providers may have with identifying and treating behavioral health issues. They also serve as a lliason with speciality behavior health. They can decrease the number of referrals of individuals automatically referred to specialty behavioral health by intervening early in the clinic. IBHCs can also assist PCMS in identifying less obvious behavioral health issues that may be interfering with effective treatment of medical illness. (MEDCOM/OTSG, IBHC manual, 2014).

IBHCs also improve access to behavioral health interventions. In the military, specialty behavioral health has traditionally been available to active duty service members and open to family members/retirees depending on availability. Providing behavioral health interventions in primary care improves access, saves cost, ensures continuity of care and empowers the PCM.

IBHCs are vital to providing early intervention. Many patients who are referred to a specialist never make it to their first appointment; thus, the PCBH model delivers care at the point of entry in a less stigmatizing fashion. This model is being implemented in the Army and the Navy; the Air Force already incorporated their version of PCBH, the Behavioral Health Optimization Program (BHOP), several years ago (Dobmeyer, 2013).

The PCBH model in the Army at this time is focused on adult primary care clinics, and these clinics provide screening for behavioral health disorders at regular intervals. Primary care providers review behavioral health screening forms for depression (Screened with PHQ-2), Anxiety (GAD-2), PTSD (PCL-4) and alcohol disorders (AUDIT-C) (MEDCOM/OTSG, IBHC manual, 2014). Primary care providers discuss positive screens with the patient, and then the primary care provider refers this patient to the IBHC. If the PCM feels a psychotropic medication is indicated, they can also consult with the External Behavioral Health Consultant (EBHC). The EBHC is a Psychiatric Advance Practice Nurse or Psychiatrist who is part of the speciality behavioral health clinic. The provider should be accessible/willing to engage with primary care as needed. See Figure 10.4.

Behavioral Health Care Facilitators (BHCF) are care facilitators that serve the adult population of the primary care clinic. A BHCF is a registered nurse who may or may not have behavioral training (MEDCOM/OTSG, IBHC manual, 2014). BHCF responsibilities include care management at either the PCM or IBHC's request. The BHCF's primary focus is on facilitating care for patients with depression, PTSD, anxiety problems or alcohol misuse (MEDCOM/OTSG, IBHC manual, 2014). BHCFs monitor patients' adherence to medications and treatment plans by following up with identified patients via phone or secure messaging and using standardized screening and program evaluation tools appropriate for the primary care population (MEDCOM/OTSG, IBHC manual, 2014).

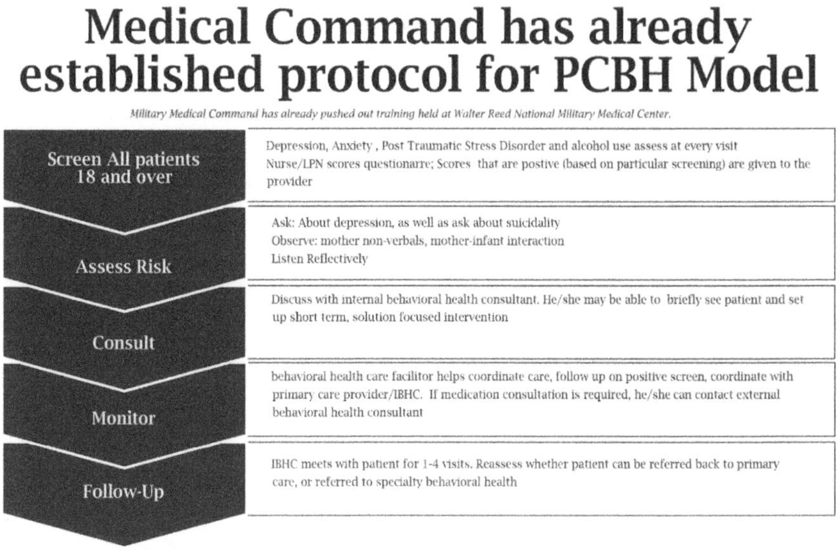

Figure 10.4 Process Diagram of Primary Care Behavioral Health

*Adapted from MEDCOM/OTSG (2014). Army Primary Care Behavioral Health (PCBH). *Internal Behavioral Health Consultant Practice Manual,* Version 2.0 retrieved from https://mitc.amedd.army.mil/sites/Communities/APCMHC/Pages/default.aspx

Collaborative Care: Child and Family Behavioral Health Services (CAFBHS)

While PCBH is an integrated care program based out of primary care, another program that has been initiated is Child and Family Behavioral Health Service (CAFBHS), which is an integrated care service that stems from behavioral health (compared to PCBH model that has roots in primary care). CAFBHS was developed because it is well recognized that there is a nation-wide shortage of pediatric behavioral health providers and difficulty accessing care for children and adolescents (MEDCOM/OTSG, 2014, Operations Order 14-44). Some military treatment facilities did not have a child psychiatrist anywhere close, or if they did, the child psychiatrist might not have been accepting patients. Similar to the PCBH program, CAFBHS collaborates with primary care clinics—both family medicine and pediatrics—to provide treatment for children and adolescents (Faran, Johnson, Ban, Shue, & Weist, 2015). Like PCBH, the CAFBHS model encourages treatment to remain in primary care as much as possible, but still have availability for consultation with specialty behavioral health (Faran et al., 2015). See Figure 10.5.

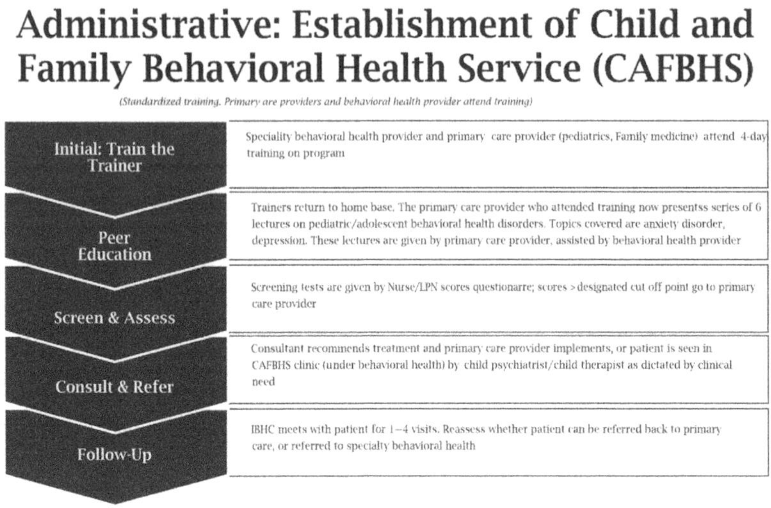

Figure 10.5 Process Diagram of Child and Family Behavioral Health System

*Adapted from MEDCOM/OTSG (2014), *Child and Family Behavioral Health System Operations Manual.* 5 February 2014. U.S. Army Medical Command, Joint Base San Antonio, TX 78234. Retrieved from: https://info.health.mil/army/bhsl/Policy/Library/OPORDsFragos. OPORD 14-44, Annex A

CAFBHS was developed in recognition that needs of family members and children are pertinent to soldier readiness (Faran et al., 2015). CAFBHS strives for standardized education and has created standardized training programs for primary care providers and behavioral health clinicians to address the most common issues in child and adolescent behavioral health: depression, anxiety and ADHD. CAFBHS has a significant emphasis on telehealth and consultation with child behavioral health providers who have dedicated time to provide specialty behavioral health care, as well as an important amount of consultation (Faran et al., 2015). Another area that CAFBHS has expanded is implementing programs by collaborating with school behavioral health programs of on-post schools. Due to resource limitations, school behavioral health is not widely implemented like the rest of program and usually requires Army bases to have a specific population/number of schools (Faran et al., 2015). CAFBHS continues to grow in its capabilities, and has sought to ensure quality of care by creating an Evidence-Based Practices curriculum that will be standardized across military treatment facilities (MEDCOM/OTSG, 2014, *Child and Family Behavioral Health System Operations Manual*).

References

American Academy of Pediatrics. (2011). *Policy Statement: Screening for Postpartum Depression at Well-Child Visits.* Los Angeles: LA Best Babies Network.

Boukydis, Z. (2012). *Collaborative Consultation with Parents and Infants in the Perinatal Period.* Budapest, Hungary: Paul Brooks Publishing.

Dobmeyer, A. (2013). Primary care behavioral health: Ethical issues in military settings. *Families, Systems, & Health, 31*(1), 60–68.

Earls, M. F., Committee on Psychosocial Aspects of Child and Family Health American Academy (2010). Incorporating recognition and management of perinatal and postpartum depression into pediatric practice. *Pediatrics, 126*(5), 1032–1039. doi:10.1542/peds.2010–2348

Faran, M., Johnson, P., Ban, P., Shue, T., & Weist, M. (2015). The evolution of a school behavioral health model in the US army. *Child Adolescent Psychiatric Clinics of North America, 24*, 415–428.

Fleming, J. W. (1996). Bright futures: Guidelines for health supervision of children. *MCN The American Journal of Maternal Child Nursing, 21*(6), 269–270. PMID: 8952277

Haworth, K. (2013). *A Pediatrician's Perspective on Postpartum Depression Screening.* Powerpoint presentation presented at the 25th Annual Postpartum Support International Conference" Whole Care for the Whole Family, Seattle, WA.

Liberto, T. (2012). Screening for depression and help-seeking in postpartum women during well-baby pediatric visits: An integrated review. *Journal of Pediatric Health Care, 26*(2). doi:10.1016/j.pedhc.2010.06.012

Lofrumento, M. A. (2008). The pediatrician's role in identifying postpartum mood disorders. In S. Stone & A. Menken (Eds.), *Perinatal and Postpartum Mood Disorders: Perspective and Treatment Guide for the Health Care Practitioner* [E-Reader Version]. New York: Springer Publishing Company, LLC.

MEDCOM/OTSG. (2014). Army Primary Care Behavioral Health (PCBH). *Internal Behavioral Health Consultant Practice Manual*, Version 2.0. Retrieved from https://mitc.amedd.army.mil/sites/Communities/APCMHC/Pages/default.aspx

MEDCOM/OTSG. (2014). *Child and Family Behavioral Health System Operations Manual.* 5 February 2014. U.S. Army Medical Command, Joint Base San Antonio, TX 78234. Retrieved from https://info.health.mil/army/bhsl/Policy/Library/OPORDsFragos. OPORD 14-44, Annex A.

Shea, S. C. (1998). *Psychiatric interviewing: The art of understanding a practical guide for psychiatrists, psychologists, counselors, social workers, nurses, and other mental health professionals* (2nd ed.). Philadelphia, PA: Saunders.

Talmi, A., Stafford, B., & Buchholz, M. (May, 2009). Providing perinatal mental health services in pediatric primary care. *Zero to Three, 29*(5), 10–16. Retrieved from https://www.zerotothree.org/resources/series/zero-to-three-journal

Chapter 11

Military Perinatal Mental Health Treatment in Behavioral Health

Ashley Clark, Nicole Champagne, and Melinda A. Thiam

Military Behavioral Health: Two Models

Introduction

Despite the numerous studies that identify the prevalence/incidence of perinatal mood and anxiety disorders present in the military population, and unlike studies published from obstetrics/prenatal care, there have been no published studies coming from the field of behavioral health. Below are two behavioral health treatment models that have been started in a military population.

A Perinatal Support Group: National Medical Center, San Diego

Ashley Clark and Nicole Champagne

General/Background

Although pregnancy has typically been considered a time of emotional well-being, studies suggest that perinatal mood and anxiety disorders (PMADs) are often the most underdiagnosed, underreported and undertreated complications of childbirth. PMADs are serious illnesses that can have a significant and lasting impact on the patient, infant and family, especially within the military population. Psychosocial perinatal support programs have been promoted to improve knowledge, attitudes and skills related to maternal mental health, but there is little known about the effects of such a support group in the military population.

Naval Medical Center San Diego (NMCSD) is the largest and most comprehensive military health care system in the Western United States. It consists of a premier teaching hospital and referral center for the Armed Forces as well as nine primary care sites for family members and eight medical clinics serving active duty personnel. In 2014, there were more than 1.2 million outpatient visits, greater than 19,000 patients admitted, and nearly 3,600 babies delivered (Spooner, Rastle, & Elmore, 2012). The Social Work Department offers classes for pregnant females, including "ABC's of Having a Military Baby" and "Single and Pregnant Active Duty." The Pediatric Department offers "Boot Camp for New Dads," "Sibling Class" and "Mom's Survival Training." The OB/GYN Department conducts labor and delivery tours when women are 32 weeks. Likewise, the Mental Health Department offers various groups for anxiety and depressive disorders. However, between these departments, there was no overlapping group to support the unique population of perinatal women with mental health disorders. Therefore, in a collaborative effort between departments, the Perinatal Support Group was formed.

A support group for postpartum depression is often more effective than a generic mothers' support group. Most mothers with PMADs feel isolated and have increased anxiety when attending a general moms' group as opposed to a program specifically designed for mothers who are suffering from mental health issues. The goal when establishing this group was to provide a safe place where struggling mothers could share their experiences with support and reassurance, while also obtaining important psychoeducation and resources.

Logistics

The Perinatal Support Group was established in 2012 as a collaborative effort between Mental Health, represented by Ashley Clark, M.D., a staff psychiatrist specializing in Reproductive Mental Health, and Obstetrics/Gynecology, represented by Nicole Champagne, LCSW. The group meets every Tuesday for an hour at the Naval Training Center (NTC), one of the outlying clinics attached to NMCSD. Patients are typically referred by providers from Mental Health, OB/GYN, or Pediatrics. Participation in the group includes females who are pregnant or up to 1-year postpartum and is open to active duty females as well as dependent spouses. Mothers are encouraged to bring in their newborns (up to 12 months) if they desire. The group is catered to new mothers who are experiencing emotional difficulties either during pregnancy, or postpartum and have symptoms that may include anxiety, excessive worries, sadness, guilt, helplessness, tearfulness, sleeping or eating problems, irritability or unwanted thoughts.

Group Structure/Format

The philosophy of the Perinatal Support Group at NTC is to create a safe space where struggling mothers can come and share their concerns and issues in a supportive environment. Each session is initiated by the introduction of the facilitators and an explanation of confidentiality. New participants fill out an intake questionnaire, and all participants fill out a weekly check-in sheet and complete an Edinburgh Postnatal Depression Scale (EPDS). The session usually begins with check-ins and updates where the participants can introduce themselves and share their struggles, positive experiences, and pose any questions to the group. The goal is to have a patient-led group where peers are supporting one another and offering validation, advice and support. The purpose of the facilitators is to moderate the discussion and provide education and clarification when needed.

Other activities are incorporated to supplement the group, including teaching sessions, guest speakers, relaxation exercises, educational videos and skills training. The LCSW provides perinatal resources for patients such as the New Parent Support Home Visitation Program; Armed Services YMCA; First 5 First Steps Home-Visiting Program, Military Outreach Ministry; Women, Infant, and Children (WIC); community Public Health visiting nurse; and the Mind-Body Medicine for Mother to be program. The Mind-Body Medicine is an evidence-based medical discipline focused on the inseparable connection between the mind and the body. The goal is for patients to develop and sustain habits for positive thoughts, emotions, and health. Mind-Body Medicine provides benefits during pregnancy such as decreased anger and irritability, the higher birthweight of newborn and decreased labor complications. Exercises from this discipline are incorporated into sessions.

The Perinatal Support Group also welcomes speakers from the programs listed above to visit the group and do short in-services on topics ranging from infant massage to purple crying to give patients an idea of the skills taught through the programs. Other guest speakers have included a child sleep specialist, a perinatal yoga instructor and a men's postpartum specialist, Daniel Singley, PhD. Dr. Singley encourages expectant dads to be involved with their partners as well as their still-in-utero baby by becoming involved early.

Results

Since starting the Perinatal Support Group in February 2012, over 140 unique patients have attended, and most attend for multiple sessions. There has been a mix of both AD women and dependents, but slightly more AD. At each visit, patients completed the EPDS. In the first year, the participants who were able to return on a regular basis showed statistically significant improvement in their posttest scores. This finding in a decrease of EPDS suggests that group therapy was an effective and beneficial treatment model to reduce symptoms of depression (Clark & Champagne, 2013).

The Perinatal Support Group has experienced a consistent stream of patients, many who attend multiple sessions. Informal feedback from the group has been positive, and many women expressed the importance of not feeling like they were alone in their emotional distress. Observationally, it was not uncommon to witness a struggling new mother improve with time to the point where she was then offering support and advice to a subsequent new mother entering the group. One participant provided written feedback stating, "It is nice being a new mom and having a support system to speak freely. It has made all the difference."

Future Directions

The Perinatal Support Group at NTC has been ongoing since February 2012, and at this time, it is a well-known resource for the community. The ultimate goal is to ensure that this group is ongoing, and therefore, it will be significant to train other providers working in the social work and mental health departments to be able to have the skills to run such a group. The foundation of this group will always be a patient-led support group, but the facilitators are also regularly always looking to incorporate other activities and speakers to supplement the group and further the education and awareness of PMADs.

Mother–Infant Dyadic Group Therapy: Ft. Belvoir Community Hospital, Ft. Belvoir

Melinda A. Thiam

General/Background

The DC metro area has a large population of military service members, as well as multiple bases for the Army, Navy, Air Force and Marines. Originally, two separate military treatment facilities served the active duty service member and military family. The National Naval Medical Center was a large Naval Hospital, and Walter Reed Army Medical Center was an Army hospital known to be the "home of warrior care." Both Walter Reed Army Hospital and National Navel Medical Center, Bethesda, were well-recognized medical centers and were the main platforms for referral and evacuation from the deployment theater, as well as supporting the military in the greater DC area. In 2011, the congressionally mandated Base Realignment and Closure (BRAC) led to the consolidation of both military hospitals into one large, joint hospital that became Walter Reed National Military Medical Center (WRNMMC). WRNMMC is located on the original Campus of the National Naval Medical Center. In addition to the consolidation of two large hospitals, DeWitt Medical Center, a small hospital at Ft. Belvoir (Alexandria, Virginia), was enlarged to become Fort Belvoir Community Hospital (FBCH).

Defining a Problem

Although WRNMMC and FBCH had a wealth of specialty and subspecialty care, there was still limited availability of behavioral health due to larger demand for services than available providers. Due to demand, priority of treatment went to active duty service members while family members as retirees were seen in military facility if space was available. Military dependent spouses with perinatal distress during or after pregnancy often struggled to obtain access to needed care as well and found limited availability of qualified professionals in the network who were comfortable treating perinatal mental illness. Due to such barriers, some mothers in crisis resorted to seeking treatment in the emergency room.

Measure

Many primary care providers screen for depression, but not always specifically perinatal depression. When perinatal depression is identified, providers can readily place a referral in the system, but unfortunately many patients who are referred to the network never make it to their first appointment. Active duty members who were referred to the behavioral clinic were booked with the next available provider, dependent on who had the nearest availability. See Figure 11.1 for the process from screening to diagnosis and treatment.

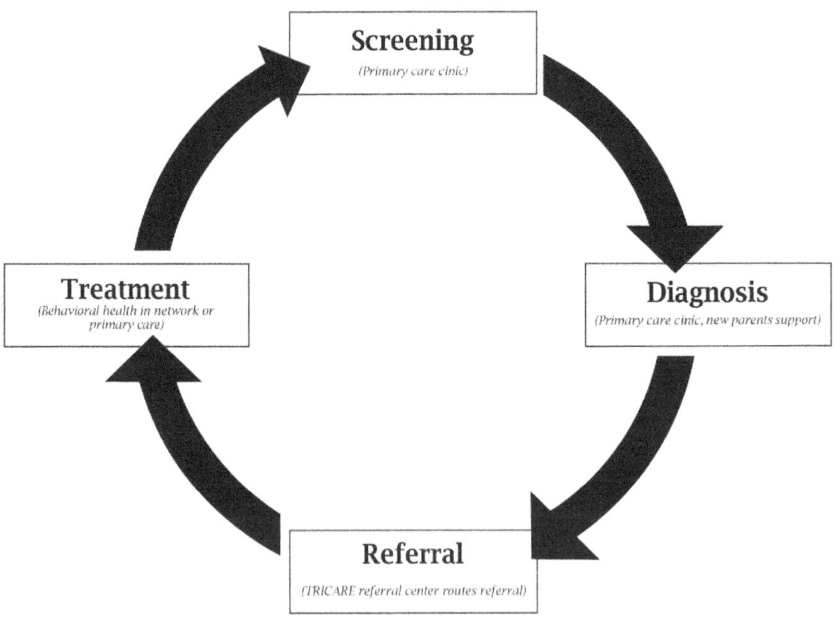

Figure 11.1 From Screening to Treatment

*Adapted from Lean Six Sigma model.

Table 11.1 Challenges Identified in Access to Care

Population baseline challenges	**Limited social support**, young age, geographical separations, logistical challenges of location in DC metro area.
Screening	No standardized screening process
Referral	**Dependent spouses wanted to be seen in the military system**, referred to network
	Limited number of available providers in network
	Network providers not comfortable/willing to treat pregnant/breastfeeding women
Treatment	**Treatment did not address mother–infant relationship**
	Unsure about quality of network care

Analyze

The behavioral health departments at both WRNMMC and FBCH recognized the need to treat both active duty military mothers and military spouses for perinatal depression, but they had limited access for pharmacological or psychological treatments for a family member. At Fort Belvoir, there was one exception to the restriction on behavioral health treatment: Although *individual* treatments were prioritized to active duty service members, *group therapy* was open to both active duty military and military spouses.

Improve

Because group therapy created an avenue for access to care, the improvement process was focused on utilizing group therapy as a treatment intervention and a means to improve access to care.

Group therapy has been found to be an effective and beneficial treatment for perinatal depression (COPE guidelines, 2011; Goodman, & Santangelo, 2011; Williams, 2014). When designing the format for the group, it was acknowledged that evidence-based literature identified that, although group therapy for perinatal depression could help ameliorate the mother's symptoms, only treating the mother would not improve the mother–infant relationship in the long term (Forman et al., 2007; Kumar & Hipwell, 1996). Fortunately, Clark, Tluczek, and Brown (2008) had published results of a pilot model for mother–infant group therapy (M-ITG) that is described in greater detail in Chapter 7. In the Clark et al. (2008) model, mothers met for 8 weekly 90-minute sessions only with other mothers, while their infants had a separate but concurrent 90-minute evaluation conducted by an infant mental health specialist. After the initial 90 minutes, mothers and infants were brought together for another 30 minutes (Clark et al., 2008).

Clark et al.'s model was too resource intense for replication in the military setting. Given the desire to use both mother–infant therapy and group therapy, Clark et al.'s model was adapted for use in a military setting and became an evidence utilization project.

Dr. Melinda Thiam, then a third psychiatry resident, designed a curriculum for a mother–infant group that was based off a modified version of Clark et al.'s (2008) pilot M-ITG model. The purpose of the group was to see if it could be a feasible and effective treatment modality to implement in a military setting. The group was designed as an open-ended group (no defined number of sessions) that were 90 minutes in length, where the entire time mothers were with their infant. Instead of a trained infant mental health specialist, both Dr. Thiam and her co-facilitator used observations skills to watch how mothers interacted with their infants and provided some assistance with addressing mother–infant relationships.

The ideal group member was identified as a new mom, at least 18 years old, who was within 12 weeks of delivery and having challenges with adjusting to new motherhood. Mothers were not required to have any diagnosable mental health disorder. Although all group participants were screened/triaged before the attending group, due to limited resources, mothers were not given any objective screening measures. See Figures 11.2 and 11.3.

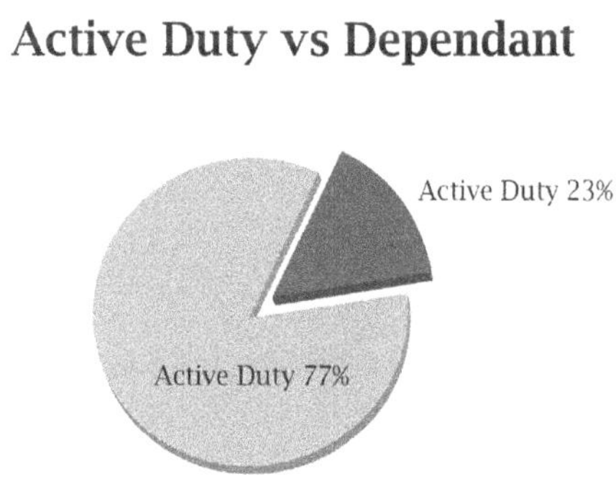

Figure 11.2 Active Duty vs. Dependent

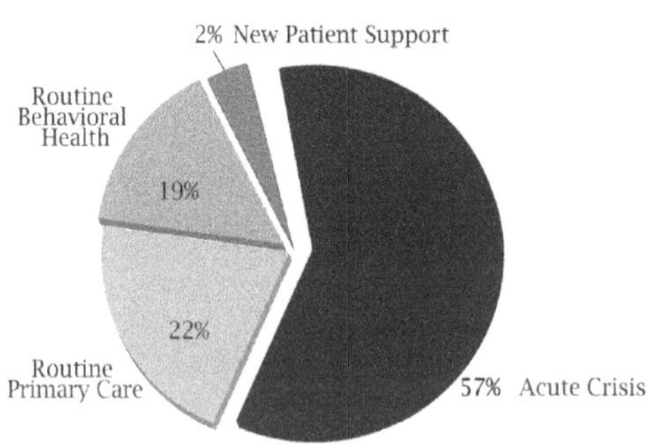

Figure 11.3 Referral Source

*Figures 11.2 and 11.3 were presented on a resident poster at the annual meeting for the American Psychological Association, May 4–7, 2014, in New York, NY.

Because most postpartum difficulties are first identified in primary care, initial collaboration was sought through reaching out to primary care clinics at both FBCH and WRNMMC. The FBCH mother–baby postpartum ward distributed the group flyer to all new mothers as part of standard postpartum education and discharge paperwork. The Army Community Service office at Ft. Meyer also advertised to groups in their publication called *Life YOUniversity*. Life YOUniversity was a newsletter that identified all small groups/educational groups and classes that are held at the various military bases in the NCR.

The psychiatry consult liaison service at Fort Belvoir facilitated many referrals from dependent mothers that they saw in the ER or that they saw at the specific request of primary care providers. The recruitment flyer was also distributed to both adult and child behavioral health departments at both Walter Reed National Military Medical Center and Fort Belvoir.

Results

The Mother–Infant Group psychotherapy group was hosted in Fort Belvoir Community Hospital (FBCH) Adult Behavior Health Clinic every Tuesday for a 90-minute block from 1600 to 1730. The first meeting started September 11, 2012, with four mothers, but subsequently became a very popular treatment modality. Within the first 18 months, there were over 44 referrals to group and over 65 group therapy sessions. Approximately 57% of referrals came from an acute setting such as FBCH Acute walk-in clinic, emergency room, Family Advocacy/Child service referral and mother–infant ward. See Figure 11.4.

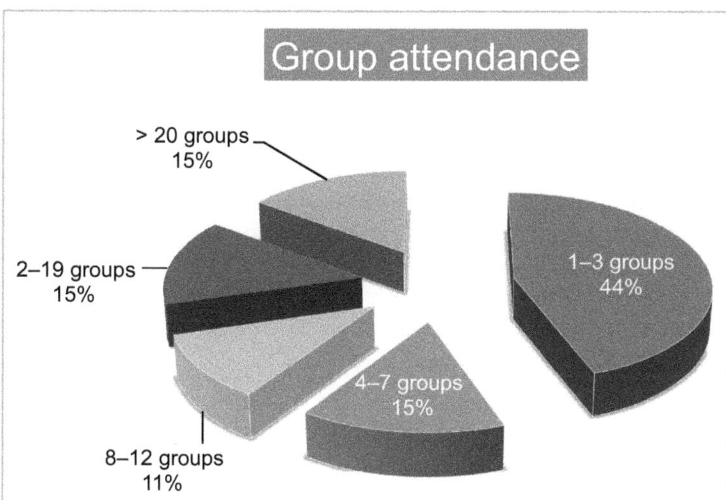

Figure 11.4 Average Group Sessions Attended

*Figure 11.4 was presented on a resident poster at the annual meeting for the American Psychological Association, May 4–7, 2014, in New York, NY.

Although no objective data were gathered, there were observable changes in the mother–infant pairs. To our knowledge, there have been no negative outcomes, and mothers who did not like or appreciate the group format did not return for a future session. Initially, the group started with more education addressing three main areas: maternal mental and physical health, infant mental health, and attachment. However, early in group development, the group format evolved into an interpersonal and process group. Themes and discussions during group sessions included discussions about the challenges of motherhood, challenges of military families, discussions about mothers' insecurities about their job as a mother, insecurities about infant feeding practices. Relationship themes included discussing marital challenges associated with having an infant, communication challenges as well as conflict with in-laws and extended family members.

One of the most enjoyable aspects of the group was discussing and observing the different mother–infant interactions within the group. The curriculum was flexible so individual mother–infant interaction could be addressed "in-the-moment" in the group. Mothers were able to state verbally their perceptions of their infants' emotional expressions and affects and would engage in nonverbal affective attunement and mirroring with their infants. When infants would become fussy, mothers were prompted to consider what crying meant to them and were able to apply practical different strategies to reduce their anxiety to soothe the infant. Facilitators and group participants alike would acknowledge and validate positive observed mother–infant interaction.

Although initially it was mainly the group facilitator verbalizing/validating observations, eventually the group transitioned to a point where other mothers were also able to validate each other and comment on mother–infant interactions that occurred within the group. Mothers frequently expressed that they enjoyed the group, and that it was a place they could be "themselves" without having to worry about what others thought of them. One particular mother was especially challenged in the beginning as she had no relationship with her mother and was in significant need of modeling. During the group, she was very attentive to other mothers interacting with their infants and used such interactions to guide her behavior. Another mother expressed "I love coming to the group and watching all of you with your children . . . it encourages me to interact more with my children and become a better mother."

Future Directions

Perinatal depression can negatively impact the health and welfare of a mother, infant, partner as well as the community. Fort Belvoir Community Hospital Adult Behavioral Health was able to successfully implement an effective and beneficial treatment modality to provide treatment to a population that was

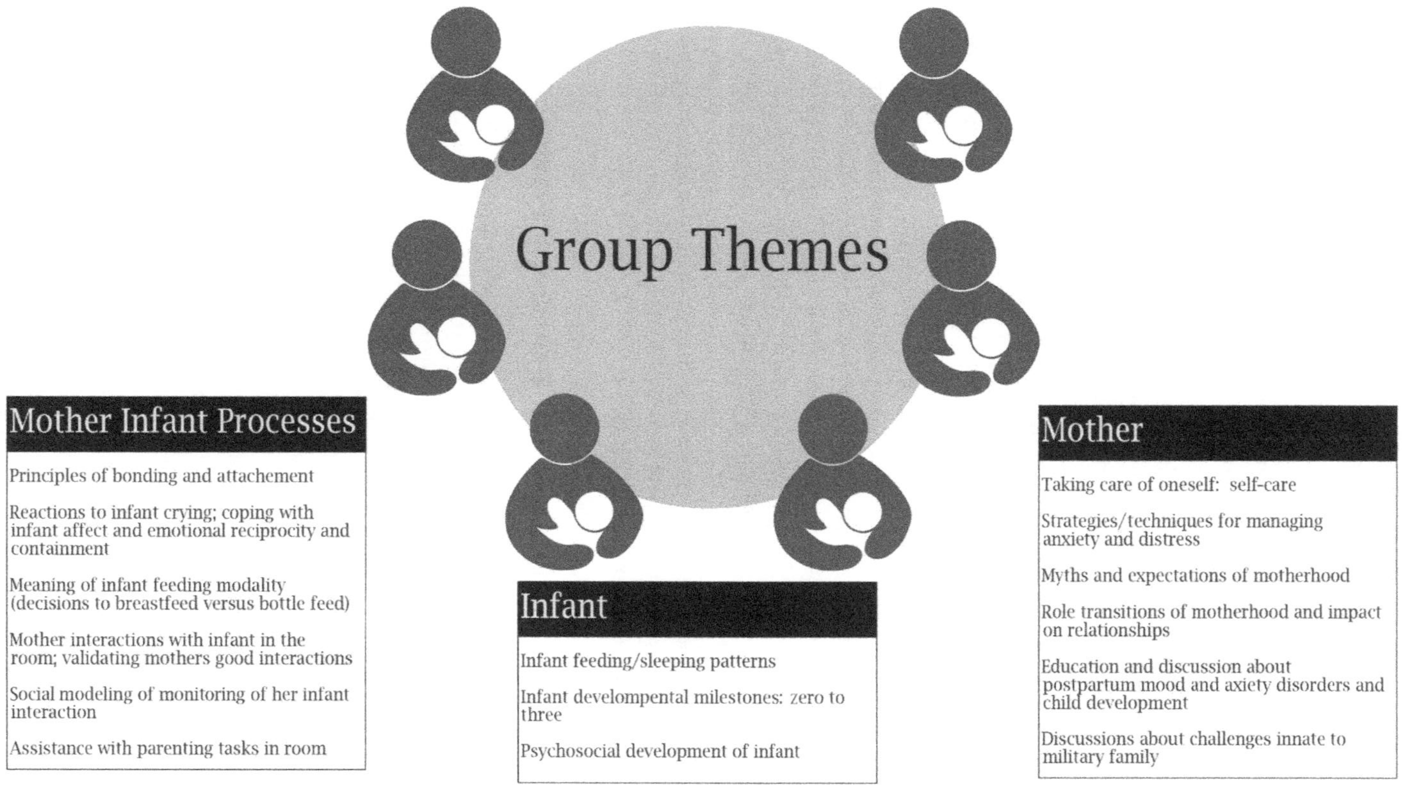

Figure 11.5 Group Therapy Themes

previously unable to receive treatment at the clinic. Additionally, Fort Belvoir was able to find that the mother–infant dyadic group model improved access to care for dependent military mothers, addressed and facilitated the mother–infant relationship and served as a supportive environment where mothers felt validated and supported by other mothers. The group design did not require extensive resources or expertise. In fact, this group was designed and started by a psychiatric resident, co-facilitated by the clinical social worker, and carried out in a general behavior health clinic in a community hospital setting.

The greatest shortcoming of this project is that it is not formal research, and we did not have any measurable outcomes. Other challenges that frequently prevented mothers from coming to the group included lack of available childcare for other children, conflicting work schedules as well as distance to the group. Several referred mothers lived up near Fort Meade or down near Stafford, Virginia, and hence, attendance required over 1 hour in DC area traffic.

The results of this evidence utilization project create the potential for military behavioral health to create a psychotherapy model and curriculum that could be standardized and implemented in standard clinical care as a treatment in military hospitals in the continental United States and overseas. A mother–infant group therapy group could be hosted by a standard behavior health clinic and well incorporated into primary care clinics or the Child and Behavioral Health service that was discussed in the previous chapter. Future goals include creating a therapy treatment manual and training module that can help guide behavioral health providers in the process of starting and continuing a mother–infant group.

Integrated Primary Care and Behavioral Health

The one unique population that is not specifically captured either in the PCBH model or the CAFBHS model discussed in the previous chapter is the pregnant and postpartum population. Pregnant and postpartum mothers are often seen in primary care clinics, especially since many bases have limited or no on base obstetric care. As seen in Dr. Elmore's project at Camp Pendleton and Dr. Haworth's work with the pediatric population, perinatal specific screening could be incorporated into primary care. In the PCBH model, primary care providers treating the mother could utilize the Edinburgh Postpartum Depression Scale for pregnant/postpartum active duty mothers. Clinic case managers could assist primary providers with positive screens by connecting with appropriated services. Internal behavioral health providers embedded in primary care clinics could provide brief, solution-focused therapy for pregnant/postpartum moms (Spooner et al., 2012) and be a link to obtain specialty behavior treatment when necessary.

CAFBHS screening could incorporate EPDS to be administered in a Well-Child Clinic, and also work with case managers to help with positive screens. Specialty behavioral health could consult with primary care physicians regarding medication. Postpartum Support International (PSI) provides certificate training presented as a multi-disciplinary approach with experienced faculty who are experienced working with a perinatal population (Indman, Meyer, & Davis, 2013). CAFBHS could utilize a program similar to PSI to provide standardized training like they have with general CAFBHS topics to train primary care and behavioral health care providers in treating this unique population. A mother–infant support group as described in San Diego or mother–infant group at Belvoir could be hosted either by the CAFBHS clinic or implemented in a primary care setting with assistance from specialty behavioral health providers.

References

BeyondBlue. (2011). Clinical Practice Guidelines (COPE): Depression and Related Disorders—Anxiety, Bipolar Disorder and Puerperal Psychosis—in the Perinatal Period: A Guidelines for Primary Care Health Professionals. Australian Government: National Health and Medical Research Counsel. Retrieved from www.beyondblue.org.au

Clark, A. L., & Champagne, N. (2013). *Effectiveness of a Perinatal Support Group in a Military Population.* American Psychiatric Association Annual Meeting; 2013 May 18–22; San Francisco, CA. Abstract NR4–17.

Clark, R., Tluczek, A., & Brown, R. (2008). A mother-infant therapy group model for postpartum depression. *Infant Mental Health Journal, 29*(5), 514–536. doi:10.1002/imhj.20189

DeLeo, B., & Waynick, T. (2014, July 30). Family life chaplains, part 1: The creation of the family life program. Retrieved from http://www.army.mil/article/130835/Family_Life_Chaplains_over_40_years_of_service_to_the_Army_Family_Part_I

Forman, D. R., O'Hara, M. W., Stuart, S., Gorman, L. L., Larsen, K. E., & Coy, K. C. (2007). Effective treatment for postpartum depression is not sufficient to improve the developing mother-child relationship. *Development and Psychopathology, 19*(2), 585–602. doi:10.1017/s0954579407070289

Goodman, J., & Santangelo, G. (2011). Group treatment for postpartum depression: A systematic review. *Archives of Women's Mental Health, 14*, 277–293. doi:10.1007/s00737-011-0225-3

Indman, P., Meyer, B., & Davis, W. (2013). *Perinatal Mood and Anxiety Disorders: Components of Care. Postpartum Support International (PSI) Pre-Conference Certificate Training.* Presented two days prior to 26th Annual Conference: Innovation and Advocacy to Support the Mental Health of Pregnant and Postpartum Families, Minneapolis, MN.

Kumar, R., & Hipwell, A. (1996). Development of a clinical rating scale to assess mother-infant interaction in a psychiatric mother and baby unit. *BJP, 169*, 18–26.

National Fatherhood Initiative. (2015). About National Fatherhood Initiative. Retrieved from http://www.fatherhood.org/about

Spooner, S., Rastle, M., & Elmore, K. (2012). Maternal depression screening during prenatal and postpartum care at a navy and marine corps military treatment facility. *Military Medicine, 177*(10), 1208–1211. Retrieved from https://www.ncbi.nlm.nih.gov/pubmed/23113449

Williams, J. (2014). Best practice guidelines for mental health disorders in the perinatal period. *BC Mental Health.* Retrieved from http://www.perinatalservicesbc.ca/health-professionals/guidelines-standards/maternal (Accessed on 24 January, 2016).

Chapter 12

Support Services in Civilian and Military Communities

Sondra S. Thompson and Melinda A. Thiam

Military awareness and services for mental and behavioral health continue to increase, but specialized treatment options for perinatal mood disorders remain underdeveloped in the military system. Therefore, much of any perinatal care and especially for specialized care such as for perinatal mood disorders is deferred to civilian network providers for military members and their families. Understanding the services locally as well as nationally is crucial in ensuring that these families are aware of all services available, both preventative and treatment.

Medical Treatment/Counseling Services

Behavioral health treatment for military members is usually available at military treatment facilities, or otherwise abbreviated as MTF. However, depending on the military installation's resources, most of this treatment is only available to the active duty service member.

TRICARE Healthcare Network

Given limited treatment availability in the military system, most family members are referred to TRICARE network providers. Although available therapists trained specifically in perinatal disorders are limited, most therapists can successfully treat a mother utilizing common therapeutic techniques and principles. While talk therapy is more available, should a woman in the perinatal period require pharmacological treatment, there seems to be a much greater disparity in resources.

Military Non-medical Counseling

Military Family Life Consultants (MFLC)

The Military Family Life Consultant Program began as a behavioral health subsidiary of Health Net, Inc. Military Family Life Consultants are trained, masters level therapists who provide short-term, non-medical counseling at military installations, during drill weekends for National Guard and Reserve members, and wherever military families come together for support—nationwide and overseas. Through the Department of Defense's Military & Family Life Counselor (MFLC) Program, there are more than 250 counselors assisting the needs of active duty, National Guard, and Reserve members, and their families with everyday issues.

Chaplain-Counseling Services

Chaplains are well known for their spiritual and religious support to the operational military. Perhaps less known about chaplain services for military families are their strong support initiatives through the chaplain's Family Life Program. Family Life chaplains have specialized education and training in counseling. Family Life chaplains are usually mid-career chaplains who have completed a second master's degree program in counseling, as well as 300 supervised practicum hours in individual and family counseling (DeLeo & Waynick, 2014). Additionally, many pursue credentials through exam and licensure to become Licensed Practical Counselors (LPCs) or Licensed Marriage and Family Therapists (LMFTs) (DeLeo & Waynick, 2015).

Chaplains are allowed the special status to provide privileged communication under the military justice system. Because of this special status allowed for military chaplains in pastoral counseling, they are uniquely suited to assist military families through difficulties of deployment stresses as well as family adjustments. Thus, the chaplains offer confidentiality in counseling soldiers and families while assisting them in some of the most difficult situations. Being able to establish a confidential trusting relationship allows chaplains to be readily available for support of military members. The chaplains work closely to coordinate with providers and other support services encouraging soldiers to seek help for needs through all available resources (DeLeo & Waynick, 2014).

Military OneSource

Military OneSource (MOS) is a website dedicated to addressing needs of service members and their families. As part of recognizing these needs, MOS has resources devoted to treating the needs of service members and their families. Titled "non-medical counseling," Military OneSource maintains a list of providers who offer free, confidential counseling that can be conducted through three main mediums: face-to-face, telephonically and online (Military OneSource, 2015). Military OneSource providers offer confidential non-medical counseling that is designed to provide short-term, goal-oriented counseling for issues that can effectively be addressed in 12 sessions, such as communication issues, adjustment to situational stressors, stress management, decision making, grief, blended-family issues and parenting skills issues. It is available for up to 12 sessions per issue, per eligible family member. Which means that someone could receive 12 sessions for one issue, perhaps something like adjusting to a deployment alone, and then, once those sessions are completed, 12 more sessions for couples-communication issues that may be experienced when the service member returns from deployment.

Key Points (Military OneSource, 2015)

- Contacts with Military OneSource, whether by telephone, online or face-to-face non-medical counseling, are private.
- Military OneSource ensures that personal information is secure, and each user is treated confidentially and with respect, regardless of rank.
- Neither service members nor their commanders are advised when a family member seeks Military OneSource non-medical counseling.
- Privacy exceptions include suspected family maltreatment (for example, domestic violence, child or elder abuse or neglect), threats to harm self or others and illegal activities. In these cases, Military OneSource consultants have a duty to report to the appropriate military and civilian authorities. Face-to-face counselors are an extension of Military OneSource, so these reporting requirements apply to them as well.

The following information obtained from the listed websites is for information purposes and in some cases, the information is taken directly from the explanations provided by the organization listed. Information is not original to this author and is provided for explanatory purposes only.

Military Programs Specific to Young Families

Family Advocacy Program

The mission of the Family Advocacy Program (FAP) is to prevent child and domestic abuse by offering programs to put a stop to domestic abuse before it starts (Military OneSource, 2015, "The Family Advocacy Program"). When abuse does occur, the FAP works to ensure the safety of victims and helps military families overcome the effects of violence and change destructive behavior patterns. The FAP also has many preventive services. These include classes/workshops on various topics such as couples' communication, anger management, stress management, effective parenting, and conflict resolution. Likewise, if a family becomes at risk for domestic violence, counseling services are available. Counseling through FAP focuses on assisting individuals and couples to understand and change attitudes, impulses, and patterns of interacting that contribute to hurtful and potentially violent behavior. The Family Advocacy Program includes specific additional programs of the New Parents Support Program and the Victims Advocacy Program (Military OneSource, 2015, "The Family Advocacy Program").

New Parents Support Program

New Parents Support Program (NPSP) is a secondary prevention program that falls under FAP as a means to prevent child abuse and neglect (Military OneSource, 2015). NPSP reaches out to families that are both expecting and/or families with children ages 0 to 3. NPSP is a federal DoD Program and thus is recognized for all military services. NPSP goals are to assist families in building strong, healthy bonds with infants/toddlers, manage the demands of parenting, help families in creating strong support networks and teach families how to interact and respond to infant and toddler behavior (Military OneSource, 2015).

The NPSP has both education classes on the post, as well as outreach services where trained providers will travel to service members' homes (on a military base or off) and teach/observe interaction with infant and toddlers. During these visits, a family member is taught parenting basics, infant interaction, different ways to bond with an infant (such as infant massage) and caring for an infant or child. The NPSP hosts playgroups/educational classes and provides families with a wealth of resources (New Parent Support Program [NPSP], 2012).

Families with more intense needs may require coordination of more intensive services. These families are followed more closely with frequent home visits, coordinated with other support agencies and sometimes engaged with FAP providers to assist and follow-up on status.

The New Parent Support Program's staff consists of nurses, social workers or home visitation specialists, and is supervised and monitored at the installation level by the Family Advocacy Program manager (NPSP, 2012; "The New Parents Support Program," 2015). The program focuses on providing one-on-one support for new and expectant parents through home visits, but some installations may offer parenting classes and groups. Services vary by service branch and by installation, but they can include:

- **Home visits.** New parents may feel more comfortable asking questions and expressing concerns about parenthood, including sleep, nutrition, behavior management, breastfeeding and other concerns in the privacy of their home, and staff can assist families in finding and taking advantage of additional services that best suit the parent's needs.
- **Prenatal and parenting classes.** Prenatal classes help parents know what to expect when the baby comes home from the hospital. Topics include feeding and nutrition, bathing and preventative health care, while parenting classes teach hands-on experience for both parents of infants and toddlers to focus on a variety of parenting issues, ranging from discipline to feeding. Classes for new fathers help them adjust to life with a new baby and support them to be an active parent.
- **Playgroups.** Structured activities in program playgroups help children improve their social and motor skills. The playgroups also help new parents get to know one another and develop a support system within the military community.

The NPSP providers maintain confidentiality and participation in the program does not impact a service member's career, nor does it result in loss of custody of children. Anything shared with a program staff member is confidential, including health-related information. There is one exception to confidentiality: Under the duty to warn, the registered nurses and licensed social workers of the NPSP are obligated to report maltreatment or suspicion that a service member or spouse may harm him or herself or others.

General Community Perinatal Resources

Postpartum Support International (PSI) (www.postpartum.net)

A statement from the website of Postpartum Support International (PSI) indicates the following: PSI was founded in 1987 by Jane Honikman in Santa Barbara, California. The purpose of the organization is to increase awareness among public and professional communities about the emotional changes that women experience during pregnancy and postpartum (Postpartum Support International, 2015).

PSI headquarters are located in Portland, Oregon, and has members all over the world, including volunteer coordinators in every one of the United States and more than 36 other countries. PSI disseminates information and resources through its volunteer coordinators, website, and annual conference. Its goal is to provide current information, resources, education, and to advocate for further research and legislation to support perinatal mental health (Postpartum Support International, 2015).

Mothers of Preschoolers (MOPS)

MOPS International is dedicated to meeting the needs of every mother of preschoolers. MOPS strives to attain this vision through the local MOPS group. A MOPS group is started through a local church and often has a leadership team made up of eight key positions, although many groups start with only two or three leaders. Most MOPS groups vary in size from 10 to 200 women. MOPS groups usually meet once or twice a month and often provide childcare through the MOPPETS program (MOPS, 2015).

Postpartum Progress®

Postpartum Progress is nonprofit peer-to-peer support organization that includes a blog website to raise awareness, fight stigma and provide peer support and programming to women with maternal mental illness (Hatfield, 2016). Postpartum Progress is one of the world's most widely read blogs dedicated to maternal mental illness and has in-depth information available of common perinatal mood and anxiety disorders (Hatfield, 2016; MOPS, 2015).

National Fatherhood Initiative

The National Fatherhood Initiative® is a 501(c)3 nonprofit organization founded in 1994. (The National Fatherhood Initiative, 2015). National Fatherhood Initiative (NFI) looks beyond maternal mental health to address paternal mental health and the importance of the role of the father. Much of this was covered in Chapter 4 on psychology of fatherhood.

National Fatherhood Initiative's mission is to improve the well-being of children by increasing the proportion of children with involved, responsible and committed fathers in their lives. NFI seeks predominately to prevent negative outcomes that occur secondary to a father's absence. NFI is the leading provider of father-specific resources for each of the nation's military branches. It seeks to expand awareness of fathers being involved in military families and has resources dedicated to building family resilience, addressing deployment challenges/reintegration, emotional wellness, and preventing domestic/child abuse (National Fatherhood Initiative, 2015). NFI has developed a program called 24/7 Dad Program that teaches fathers skills of individual resilience as well as teaching skills centered around their role as a man, as a father, husband and/co-parent. (National Fatherhood Initiative, 2015).

Boot Camp for New Dads http://www.bootcampfornewdads.org/

Boot Camp workshops feature veteran dads talking frankly about their experiences as they became dads and the issues they found to be most important (Bishop, G., 2015). Each new group of veterans adds their insights, which keeps the course content fresh and focused on the real needs of new fathers.

The veteran fathers, with their babies on their laps, are very effective in communicating to other men the opportunities and rewards of personally caring for and connecting with their children (Bishop, G., 2015). Their expectations that each man will do their best for their children is implicit in everything they say and do, and their straightforward explanations of the realities they faced and their encouragement create a trusting and motivating environment (Bishop, G., 2015). Men respond to a challenge from other men, as well as to the guidance of those with experience, and the best traditions of sports and the military is represented in Boot Camp's man-to-man training approach.

Boot Camp prepares men to be dads in all respects, starting with holding and comforting a real baby (Bishop G., 2015). Veteran dads demonstrate burping, changing, swaddling, the "trouble shooter's guide" to crying babies, and deal with a broad set of issues including bonding, work hours, forming a parenting team, safety, preventing child abuse, dealing with relatives, etc. The experiences of thousands of Boot Camp veterans provide the course content, and they place the strongest emphasis on the tremendous support new moms need from dads (Bishop, A., 2015).

Boot Camp for Moms

While there are plenty of resources for moms-to-be, there aren't any that inform her of what's going on with dad and how they can bring out the best in each other when they are starting their new family this is where the Boot Camp for New Moms Program is helpful (Bishop, A., 2015). There are lots of classes that tell her what to expect during labor and delivery, but none that help her navigate the changes in her relationship and life once she brings this new little human home (Bishop, A., 2015). Boot camp for moms is traditionally conducted in a group setting wherein new mothers have opportunity to discuss, ask questions and be mentored by more experienced mom (Bishop, A., 2015).

Other Community Perinatal-Related Programs

Breastfeeding

Breastfeeding in Combat Boots www.breastfeedingcombatboots.com

This resource is a nongovernmental organization dedicated to encouraging military moms to breastfeed. This website is marketed toward active duty women and provides critical information/resources for active duty mothers on various topics involved with breastfeeding and caring for new infants while simultaneously serving on active duty. The website has links to the different military policies on breastfeeding and actually has templates/memoradums that active duty women can use if they need to advocate for the ability to pump breast milk during duty day (Roche-Paull, 2015).

Baby Carriers

Ruckabye Baby http://ruckabyebaby.org/

Provides free baby carriers to any injured active duty, reserve or veteran service members with children under 2 years of age.

The Carrying On Project www.carryingonproject.org/

The Carrying On Project assists military families to obtain carriers and promote "babywearing" and bonding, especially for military families that are separated due to service or injuries.

Baby Showers

Military Ovation (North Dakota)—CamoKisses
http://www.militaryovation.org/families/

Showering pregnant troops, veterans or spouses with pampering moments, with a special focus on deployment pregnancies.

Operation Help a Hero
www.operationhelpahero.org/ohh-baby-showers.html

Operation Help a Hero is a public charity made up of all volunteers dedicated to the well-being and care of military members. Their programs focus on support of military units and families as they prepare to deploy, during and on their return.

Operation Homefront—Star Spangled Babies
www.operationhomefront.net

Operation Homefront provides exciting morale building opportunities through a variety of programs. One such program is Star Spangled Babies, a baby shower hosted by local Operation Homefront chapters for expectant military spouses or female service members or those about to adopt, in the paygrades of E-1 through E-6.

Operation Shower http://operationshower.org/

Operation Shower provides the experience of a baby shower for military families who are expecting a new baby and have a service member deployed or recently deployed. They provide and coordinate baby showers with emphasis on "high-quality products" provided.

Operation Showers of Appreciation http://osoamil.org/

Operation Showers of Appreciation is a nonprofit tax-exempt, volunteer, and donation-based organization, who provide gifts for newborn babies and support through hosting and co-hosting large scale baby showers for local military and their families.

San Diego Military Outreach Ministries (SDMOM)
www.sandiegomom.org

SDMOM is an incorporated charity supported by churches, civic organizations, businesses, military members and private donors working with other nonprofit organizations. SDMOM provides free helping services to thousands of enlisted families each year. Services are intended for enlisted members of ranks E-5 and below and include nearly daily distribution of food, furniture, and household goods, children's supplies and hosting holiday events, baby showers and family events.

Blankets

Operation Attachment www.operationattachment.org

Operation Attachment is a group focused on supporting bonding between deployed fathers and their newborns by providing handcrafted newborn blankets to be sent to fathers in country so they can sleep with the blankets and send them home, allowing their infants to learn their father's smell and assist with bonding.

Budget for Baby (Marines, Navy)

Budget for Baby www.nmcrs.org/pages/budgeting-for-a-baby

Available at all NMCRS locations only, The Budget for Baby program is a series of workshops conducted by volunteers to educate about the impact that a new baby can have on family finances and planning for this. Attendees receive a layette gift.

Doula

Operation Special Delivery www.operationspecialdelivery.com

Operation Special Delivery (or OSD) provides trained volunteer doulas for pregnant women whose husbands or partners have been severely injured or who have lost their lives due to the current war on terror, or who will be deployed at the time that they are due to give birth. What is a doula? A doula is specially trained to provide informational, emotional and physical support to women during childbirth. A doula does not perform medical tasks but is trained to provide sustained support to a mother in labor.

Gifts, Gift Baskets

MOM4USA www.mom4usa.org

Expectant mothers may register to receive a Baby Care Package full of essential infant items.

Operation Military Baby (Operation Helping Hand/American Angels) www.operationhelpinghand-americanangels.com/babyoutreach

Operation Military Baby ships items (hats, blankets, outfits) to Ft. Stewart, Georgia, and mail all-year-round.

Operation Top Knot (Soldiers' Angels) www.soldiersangels.org/top-knot

Top Knot is a nationwide network of service clubs and individuals who sew, knit and shop to create gift baskets for infants and expectant mothers in military families. Volunteers knit, crochet, sew, quilt, and design items for babies and provide other homemade gifts. Members also assemble and deliver gift baskets full of goodies and necessities.

Ultrasound CD-ROM

www.storkvision.com

Stork Vision® provides a free duplicate CD-ROM from the ultrasound session of all baby's pictures to expectant military mothers whose husbands are deployed or going to be deployed.

Military Family Resources

Table 12.1 Military Family Programs

Army	Soldier and Family Support Centers and Army Community Services (ACS) The mission of Army Community Service (ACS) is to • Facilitate commander's ability to provide comprehensive, coordinated and responsive services that support readiness of Soldiers, civilian employees and their families. Areas: Mobilization and Deployment Readiness and Stability and Support Operations Soldier and Family Readiness Relocation Readiness Employment Readiness Financial Readiness

(*Continued*)

Table 12.1 (Continued)

Navy	Fleet and Family Support Center (FFSC) Fleet and Family Support Programs (FFSP) support individual and family readiness through a full array of programs and resources which help Navy families to be resilient, well-informed and adaptable to the Navy environment. Programs include: • Deployment and Ombudsman support for Sailors and Their Families • Personal and Family Wellness Education and Counseling • Emergency Preparedness and Response • Crisis Intervention and Response • Military and Personal Career Development • Financial Education and Counseling • Relocation Assistance • Transition Assistance • Spouse Employment • Sexual Assault Prevention and Response • New Parent Support • Podcasts and Webinars
Air Force	Airmen and Family Readiness Center (AFRC) The Airman and Family Readiness Center serves as a one-stop information and referral center for single, married, active duty, Guard, Reserves, civilians who work on base, and retired members as well as their families. One of its major functions is linkage—ensuring Team Nellis personnel and their families are connected with the appropriate service on and off base. Relocation Services: • Personal and Family Readiness • Air Force Aid Society • Personal Financial Readiness • Personal and Work-Life Education • Exceptional Family Member Support • Volunteerism • Airman's Attic • Career Development • Transition to Civilian Life • School Liaison Officer • Casualty Assistance (located in the Military Personnel Flight, Building 20)
Marine Corps	Marine and Family Services (M & FS) Marine & Family Programs is a community-based division of MCCS that supports the individual Marine and Sailor and their families. With a knowledgeable, well-trained and experienced staff of social workers, educators and specialists, Marine & Family Programs has something for everyone from employment aid and education to counseling and childcare. The services provided by Marine and Family Programs are organized under 1 of 4 branches: Family Readiness, Family Care, Personal and Professional Development, and Behavioral Health.

Coast Guard Work-Life Center, located in each district office

Family Readiness Groups

- A peer information and referral system that passes information from the command to the family during deployments.
- Volunteers are trained to communicate professionally and know available resources.

Note: You should be sure your family readiness group has up-to-date contact information for you at all times.

- Army—Family Readiness Group (FRG)
- Navy—Ombudsman Program (OP)
- Marine Corps—Key Volunteer Network (KVN) and Lifestyle Insights Networking Knowledge Skills (LINKS)
- Air Force—Key Spouse

Finally, contact Military OneSource

Stateside: 1-800-342-9647,
Overseas: 1-800-3429-6477, or Overseas Collect: 1-484-530-5908
http://www.militaryonesource.com

- *Military OneSource Parenting Page*—The Parenting page has helpful content worth exploring. You can find great information on adoption, parenting skills and child development stages, as well tips for dealing with grief and loss, divorce, bullies, routines and discipline.
- *New Parent Support Program*—We all say we're going to read the big parenting books and learn everything we possibly can, but who has time for that with a new baby? New and expecting parents can build a network of support with the New Parent Support Program instead. Manage those first few years with access to trained staff who can answer parenting questions, provide home visits or even set you up with supervised playgroups and parenting classes.
- *Exceptional Family Member Program*—Don't go it alone. If you have a child with special needs, check out the Exceptional Family Member Program page on Military OneSource. Read a collection of articles with specific assistance and resources for military family members with special needs.
- *Military Childcare programs*—Childcare that's high quality and affordable? Yes, please. This article explains how to locate quality, affordable child care in your community, both on and off the installation.
- *Create a safe sleep environment for your infant*—The one thing all parents want more of—sleep! Find sleep again by learning how to set a bedtime routine and how to make your infant's sleeping environment safe.

Supplementary Military Programs

Military One Source—Zero to Three provides a comprehensive collection of materials for parents, caregivers and professionals who work to meet the needs of military families with babies and toddlers affected by events such as deployment and reunification. To order materials at no charge, visit Military OneSource and go to the "orderable materials" page. www.militaryonesource.mil

FOCUS: Families OverComing Under Stress—As a service initiated by the Bureau of Medicine and Surgery (BUMED), the Families OverComing Under Stress (FOCUS) Project addresses concerns related to a parent's combat operational stress injuries and combat-related physical injuries by providing family resiliency services to military children and families. www.focusproject.org/

Comprehensive Soldier and Family Fitness—Comprehensive Soldier and Family Fitness (CSF2) is designed to build resilience and enhance the performance of the Army Family—Soldiers, their Families, and Army Civilians. CSF2 does this by providing hands-on training and self-development tools. http://csf2.army.mil/about.html

Reach Out and Read—Reach Out and Read promotes early literacy and school readiness in pediatric exam rooms nationwide by giving new books to children and giving advice to parents about the importance of reading aloud. www.reachoutandread.org/

Real Warriors Campaign—The Real Warriors Campaign is an initiative launched by the Defense Centers of Excellence for Psychological Health and Traumatic Brain Injury (DCoE) to promote the processes of building resilience, facilitating recovery and supporting the reintegration of returning service members, veterans and their families.

The Real Warriors Campaign promotes help-seeking behavior among service members and veterans. www.realwarriors.net/

The Military Child Education Coalition—The Military Child Education Coalition's (MCEC) work is focused on ensuring quality educational opportunities for all military-connected children affected by mobility, family separation, and transition. MCEC performs research, develops resources, conducts professional institutes and conferences, and publishes resources for all constituencies. www.militarychild.org/

The National Military Family Association—The mission of the National Military Family Association (NMFA) is to fight for benefits and programs that strengthen and protect uniformed services families and reflect the nation's respect for their service. www.militaryfamily.org/

Uniformed Services University Center for the Study of Traumatic Stress—The work of the Center for the Study of Traumatic Stress (CSTS) addresses a broad scope of trauma exposure from the consequences of combat, operations other than war, terrorism, natural and human-made disasters, and public health threats. CSTS is a part of the nation's federal medical school, Uniformed Services University (USU), and its Department of Psychiatry, as well as a partnering center of the newly established Defense Centers of Excellence (DCoE) for Psychological Health and Traumatic Brain Injury. www.centerforthestudyoftraumaticstress.org/

United Through Reading—United Through Reading's mission is to unite families facing physical separation by facilitating the bonding experience of reading aloud together. The programs developed by United Through Reading provide opportunities for emotional bonding that relieve the stress of separation and instill a love of reading by providing the opportunity for family members to make a recording on DVD of themselves reading a book aloud to their children. www.unitedthroughreading.org/

Give an Hour—www.giveanhour.org—Give an Hour™ is a 501(c)(3) nonprofit that is a national network of mental health providers who provide free counseling and mental health treatment to military service members. Give an Hour™ is a volunteer organization wherein mental health providers provide essentially free face-to-face or telebehavioral health treatment. These providers offer counseling for individuals, couples and families, and children and adolescents. Volunteer providers also work to reduce the stigma associated with mental health by participating in and leading education, training and outreach efforts in schools and communities and around military bases.

References

Bishop, A. (2015). Boot Camp for New Moms. Retrieved from www.bootcampfornewmoms.com

Bishop, G. (2015). Boot Camp for New Dads, About us. Retrieved from www.bootcampfornewdads.org

DeLeo, B., & Waynick, T. (2014a, July 30). Family Life Chaplains, Part 1: The Creation of the Family Life Program. Retrieved from www.army.mil/article/130835/Family_

DeLeo, B., & Waynick, T. (2014b, August 4). Family Life Chaplains, Part II: Strong Bonds and Beyond. Retrieved from www.army.mil/article/131263/

DoD Issuances. (2012, June 13). Department of Defense Instruction Number 6400.05. New Parent Support Program. Retrieved from www.dtic.mil/whs/directives

Hatfield, J. (2016). About Us: Postpartum progress, what we do. Retrieved from www.postpartumprogress.org

Military OneSource. (2015). About Military OneSource. Retrieved from www.militaryonesource.mil/footer?content_id=267441

Mothers of Preschoolers International. (2015). Frequently Asked Questions. Retrieved from www.mops.org

National Fatherhood Initiative. (2015). About National Fatherhood Initiative. Retrieved from www.fatherhood.org/about

Postpartum Progess, Inc. (n.d.). Postpartum Progress, What We Do. Retrieved from www.postpartumprogress.org
Postpartum Support International. (2015). Overview: What Is Postpartum Support International (PSI). Retrieved from www.postpartum.net/about-psi/overview/
Roche-Paull, R. (2015). About Breastfeeding in Combat Boots, Founder, Mission. Retrieved from breastfeedingincombatboots.com

Other Resources of Interest

Providers Resources

Infantrisk.org
Marcesociety.com
MedEdPPD.org
Motherfriendly.org
NIMH.nih.gov
Postpartum.net
Postpartumstress.com
PSYweb.com
Womensmentalhealth.org

Peer Support, Dads and Grief

1800ppdmoms.org
Jennyslight.org
Missfoundation.org (for families who have lost a child for any reason)
Mothertobaby.org
Mommiescrytoo.com
Postpartumdads.org
Postpartummen.com
ppdsupportpage.com
Projectfamily.org
Projectfatherhood.org

Chapter 13

"In Their Own Words . . ." Survivor Stories

Amy De Nardo-Kaczmarek

Individual stories from military families written in their own words.

(For protection of privacy, no names are given)

Military Civilian Spouse Stories

United States Air Force (USAF) Spouse

I got your name from the Postpartum Support International Directory, and I wanted to reach out and say "Thank You" for your involvement in the organization. I read your poem and liked it very much. I'm a new member, a mother of two, and a postpartum psychosis survivor. Over 30 years ago, I gave birth to a premature son while my husband was overseas. My nicest Mother's Day gift ever was when that son called to say that he was back in the States after a tour of duty in Afghanistan. He was active duty Air Force at the time and is now in the Air Force Reserve. . . . My heart goes out to those mothers who give birth when their husbands are deployed, as well as to mothers who have to deploy when they have young children. It's great to know that there is someone within the military providing postpartum support to families.

Sent to Postpartum Support International

United States Air Force (USAF) Spouse

I was taken away in a straightjacket 11 days after giving birth to a premature baby on the ward of an Air Force hospital. I am sharing my story because I believe from the bottom of my heart that my postpartum psychosis was avoidable. Although it happened 35 years ago, it stands out as the worst experience of my life. As I've learned more about perinatal mood disorders, I have come to realize how fortunate I was to make a complete recovery from my psychosis. However, the experience affected my mother/child relationship and cast a long shadow of guilt and shame across my psyche that lasted over 25 years.

At the time, I was 26 years old, a college graduate, married 5 years to an Air Force pilot, and the mother of a 3-year-old son. I had no mental health complications in either my first or a subsequent third childbirth. I was working full time up until about 1 week before I started to have complications from my pregnancy. At which time, I quit my job abruptly. My husband left for a Temporary Duty (TDY) assignment to Okinawa and was scheduled to return shortly before my due date.

Neighbors took me to the base emergency room 3 times within a week. On none of these occasions was my blood pressure taken. On the first visit, I complained of abdominal discomfort and constipation and was given a strong laxative. On the second visit, I was told I was having premature labor contractions. I was checked and told to go home. On the third visit, I again complained of premature labor contractions and was sent home. At a subsequent pregnancy checkup, my blood pressure was taken; and it was 180/120. I was immediately admitted to the hospital for toxemia/preeclampsia.

On the night my son was born, I asked a nurse for a watch to time my contractions. Five minutes before my son was born prematurely in the ward, I reported that my contractions were coming every 5 minutes, and was told to go to sleep and stop bothering the nurses. I will credit an Air Force nurse and doctor with extremely prompt and calm action after they realized that I was indeed in labor. The doctor was there for the delivery and immediately took the baby to the nursery. A pediatrician was called in to care for the baby, who was 6 weeks premature and weighed 3 lbs. 9 oz.

Over the next week, I gradually learned to express my breast milk, which I did every 3 hours. There was some discussion of transporting my son to a neonatal intensive care unit at another Air Force hospital. However, my son was doing well, and I was available to provide fresh breast milk. The staff decided to keep my son and me at the hospital. As the unit was getting full, I also had a series of roommates, all who were on a four-hour feeding schedule. Between expressing my milk and vital checks, I rested but got negligible sleep. I remember being woken from a deep sleep shortly after delivering my baby, but after that, I do not believe I experienced any deep sleep for the rest of my hospital stay.

Approximately 1 week after I gave birth, my husband returned early from his TDY. We started to make plans for me to go home. We lived off base, which was a 45-minute drive away, so it would have been virtually impossible for me to go home and deliver fresh milk every 3 hours. It was 1979, and the hospital staff was not aware or did not mention the option of using a breast pump and freezing the milk.

The hospital staff began to realize I was not sleeping and was becoming mentally unstable. They encouraged me to take breaks from the hospital, go shopping at the Base Exchange (BX), and even take one night off of breastfeeding. My last roommate had Rhesus (rH) factor and had issues with her baby's health. I subsequently learned that her baby had died around the time that my psychotic break occurred. I felt the hospital staff was not giving proper medical care to my baby and me, and insisted I was leaving immediately with my baby.

I was told I could leave, but the baby had to stay. I slapped a nurse and was taken away in a straightjacket to a nearby county mental health ward.

I was released from the mental health ward to return to my home, but the following day, after a home visit, I was admitted involuntarily to the mental health ward. I refused to take medication, and five people held me down and medicated me against my will. I was in the ward for 2 weeks, and when I was allowed to go home, I could barely walk, talk or control my bladder. I was assigned to a psychiatrist and gradually weaned off of medication over a period of months. When my baby was released from the hospital, at approximately 5 weeks of age, I tried to resume breastfeeding but was unsuccessful.

I had a shaky recovery, with one relapse in which I had issues with sleep and became slightly psychotic. At that point, I was afraid of being committed to the mental ward again and discontinued psychiatric care. Fortunately, the episode resolved over time, and I made a complete recovery by one year postpartum. During that year, I struggled with poor self-esteem and an eating disorder.

I had breastfed my first son exclusively and felt that I had been the perfect mother to him, in contrast to being a very poor mother to my second son. Although I never spoke about my psychosis, I always felt I should have given my second son a better start to life. For nearly 25 years, I blamed every struggle or issue with my son on the psychosis. This was finally resolved when my son enlisted in the Air Force and became a responsible young man at age 26.

Around that same time, I started to read about maternal mental health, including the book Women's Moods. *I became involved as a volunteer in the field of maternal mental health and met other women who had experienced postpartum psychosis. I learned that postpartum psychosis is multi-factorial, and I realized my personality type, hormonal changes, and lack of social support all factored into my psychosis. I can understand now that I should have done several things differently, including having my mother come out during my hospital stay for support; instead I had asked her to wait until I came home from the hospital with my preemie.*

I believe the overwhelming factor causing my psychosis was sleep deprivation. I hope military hospitals, families, and caregivers will all give attention to the sleep status of new moms and ensure a period of uninterrupted sleep every night.

United States Army (USA) Male Civilian Spouse

When a soldier makes sacrifices, the entire family sacrifices, and this wears on you after a while. Being a spouse of an active duty soldier and a father of two is very demanding. For over 20 years, I have endured the struggles of parenthood mostly as a single parent because of my wife going on multiple deployments. These struggles consist of caring for the kids as far as meals, school and household chores, just to name a few. Another struggle is the constant Permanent Change of Station (PCS) moves, which doesn't allow you to hold down a permanent job in the civilian sector, so you have the added stress of having the military as your only option for employment.

As a man, you are always looked at as the defender of your family, but when it comes to your military wife deploying, you have to come to grips with the fact that your wife will be put in situations and areas around the world that are totally out of your control. There isn't much you can do to protect her. My wife wants to do 30 years in the military, but due to the stress of being a family member and husband of a soldier, I have come to the conclusion this is our last tour as a family because I have decided the constant moving and military life is just too much.

Speaking from my personal experience, I can tell anyone it's more frustrating to be a family member than it is to be on active duty as you are always dealing with uncertainty. Not knowing where you're going to work, where your kids will go to school, where you will live, etc. This continuous stress can eat away at a person like cancer. However, my primary goal is to make sure during each PCS or deployment, the kids are not inconvenienced. With that being said, this is our last tour as a family, and as my wife continues her career, our family is headed for something more stable and less stressful.

Military Personnel Stories

Active Duty Mother, Married to a Civilian Spouse

I had always declared I was never going to get married or join the military. I didn't want to be dual active duty, so I figured military marriage/family was never going to happen. Yet, soon in my military career, I met my husband and we soon married. Soon after marriage, we were relocated across the country to our last choice duty assignment. We had a great support network at our last duty station; now, we had next to nothing.

Within a few weeks of arrival, we discovered we were pregnant. There was both joy and a sense of fear. Joy for parenthood, but dread for how this was going to balance with my military career, especially in health care. I had to inform my residency about my pregnancy, which seemed to give others a bad first impression of me in my new work environment. I recall working 24–30hr shifts in my first trimester, and was very nauseated and feeling poor. I seemed to have contractions all throughout pregnancy. I became embarrassed and was afraid of looking like I was sandbagging it or not pulling my fair share.

Working in the medical field, there were no shortages of horror stories about new parents or mothers in labor from my colleagues. At 24 weeks, I really started struggling. By 30 weeks, I was having notable Braxton-Hicks contractions almost daily, especially after long shifts. I was eventually placed on limited call, wherein my call shifts were changed from 24–30hrs to 18–24hrs. This caused resentment in my colleagues since it meant they had to cover. I tried to push through. At 37 weeks, I had regular contractions, so I thought I was in labor. I went to triage, only to find out it wasn't labor.

I had requested duty limitation to work 6-to-8-hour days given it was hard working in a clinic with sick kids, who were often combative. The OB-resident looked at me and said, "I don't know what to tell you . . . pregnancy isn't easy. And just to let you know, my colleague went until the day before she delivered her baby still performing C-sections." I was stunned. When I went back to my supervisor, I was in tears and was about to quit the specialty. I reluctantly rescinded my resignation and tried to gut it out. Given my negative experience with OB, I stayed home, vowing I would not go to the hospital until the very last minute.

However, on my due date, I started vomiting profusely and couldn't keep food/fluid down. I still didn't want to go. Eventually, I became dehydrated and could barely walk, which resulted in having to go to the hospital via ambulance. I was dreading the insensitive comments that were sure to come once I arrived. Instead, I found out I was at 8cm, and my daughter was born within 30 minutes of reaching hospital—a brief reprieve.

Maternity leave was okay, but I held onto a sense of dread about going back to work, since I would be working with everyone else's kids, instead of being at home with my own child. That dreaded day came, and I returned to work. I hated it. I was already resentful because of the climate that ensued during pregnancy. I struggled to find time to pump and was overwhelmed managing my work I once was able to manage. My work became slower and slower. I was angry with myself for being away from my child and felt like a bad mother, who was "never home."

Starting back on call was miserable. I despised work. When I had to return to an inpatient environment, I was even more miserable. I could not maintain focus and seemed to struggle to keep up with others. I felt detached from my daughter, who now didn't even want to breastfeed when she had the opportunity—bottle only. I had to repeat clinical rotations, due to suboptimal performance. For several months, I dreaded going to work and felt my daughter was better off without me. I was too numb to think further. Eventually, I ended up resigning from this given specialty and changing career fields.

At one point, one medical provider accused me of being narcissistic, since he told me, "You intentionally became pregnant with no consideration of how it would affect your colleagues." I was again shocked at such a response. Another time, when I sought help in the military system—I was told because I had struggled with Postpartum Depression, so I should not be in the military or in the medical field and then was compared to the 2009 Fort Hood shooter. Fortunately, these comments were limited to a select number of providers and the remaining providers were helpful. Once, I was away from the toxic work environment, I was able to start to recover. I felt like I became a mother again.

I eventually had another daughter almost 3 years later. This time, the work environment was more supportive. My subsequent time in the military has always been a challenge to find balance. However, now, I can enjoy both roles. I learned others would have their opinions of me, and I could not make everyone happy. Also, to take care of others, I also had to take care of myself.

Active Duty Mother, Who Is Dual-Military

During my time in the military, I was pregnant twice. The first time I was pregnant, my husband just came back from a year deployment. I was too afraid to tell anyone about my pregnancy, especially after sitting across from my Sergeant First Class (SFC) at lunch and hearing about how female soldiers were just "getting pregnant to get out of doing their jobs." If he had only known that I was also pregnant, he might not have said how he truly felt. His words prevented me from telling him what I wanted to say since I believed he probably would have thought I went from being a stellar soldier to one of the worst soldiers in the company. At that moment, I carried on like nothing was different. For example, I did a 12-mile road march and was chosen to go to assault school as a walk-on. Unfortunately, the assault school spots were full, and I did not attend the class. However, when I finally mustered the courage to tell my SFC that I was pregnant, I miscarried that same day at almost 12 weeks.

Then, 3 months later, I was sent to assault school again. This time, I was one of two soldiers to be given a slot for my company, and I was so excited to be going. However, on day zero, during the obstacle course, I was too weak to climb the rope and failed out of the course for the first time. The next day, I had a Battalion run, and during the run, I kept falling back, but not to the point of falling out of formation. However, the change was enough for one of the medical officers in my company to take notice, so he asked me after the run if I was okay. I told him I must be weak from the obstacle course I had done the day before since I was all bruised up, or maybe, there was a possibility I was just getting sick. After we had been done talking, I thought for a moment, and it hit me. I could be pregnant again.

The next morning, I went to sick call, and sure enough, I was pregnant. My disappointment from failing out of assault school went to overwhelming joy at the idea that I was going to have another child. This time, I told the command right away. Of course afterward, my joy did not last long, since the command began treating me differently. For example, I was sitting next to another soldier when the SFC told him that I could not look better on paper than him, since I was pregnant, and we both were going to the promotion board at the same time for the same Military Occupational Specialty (MOS). This brought back all the emotions from my first pregnancy and made me feel isolated and alone.

When I was 3 months pregnant and in my second trimester, my unit sent me on a Stateside Temporary Duty Assignment (TDY) until the day I reached 5 months gestational period, since, after that, I could not travel by regulation. However, while I was on TDY, my command still treated me unfairly and took advantage of my condition. For example, the Battalion Commander called on me specifically one evening, so I thought this must be something of honor. Nope, not one bit. He had appointed me as a designated duty driver until early morning while all the other soldiers were allowed to drink alcohol at the local bar for the holiday weekend. Also, the Command sent soldiers home that were diagnosed in their first trimester. This made me furious, especially after I found out during my TDY that my husband was being deployed again overseas, so by the time I returned home, I would only have about 2 months until he deployed again.

After I had arrived home from TDY, I spent the next 2 months on a roller coaster ride of emotions. I was worried about everything to include the deployment, the pregnancy, and the command climate. Even now as a dual-military soldier, you know there is always a possibility of your military spouse being deployed. However, I was upset my husband had only been home from an overseas deployment for less than 12 months and then was attached to a unit from another state to deploy again. I did not think the process was fair. The only thing that comforted me was he did not deploy while I was TDY.

For those 2 months, we spent as much time as we could to prepare for the new baby and his upcoming deployment. Everything seemed to be happening too fast, and I knew once my husband deployed I would be on my own. I had no family living near me, and our closest family was 14 hours away or two states away. We lived 45 minutes from the Army base, so no one actually visited us, since most people thought the distance was too far, especially in bad weather.

During the last month of my pregnancy, I was bedridden, due to preeclampsia and gestational diabetes. I could not tell my husband about my situation, and no one in my unit ever came by or even called to check up on me, except one of my civilian co-workers, who was my friend. I was shocked, I could have died on my couch and no one in my command would have even known. Then, one day, a Non-Commissioned Officer (NCO) came to the door and told me my yard needed tending to since the grass needed to be cut. I was flabbergasted but had to hold my composure. I told him politely I could not cut the grass, due to being bedridden, and there was no one else to cut it since my husband was deployed. After he made a complaint about my situation to someone on the Army base, my unit finally came to my residency to cut my grass, which was the one and only time during my pregnancy and after giving birth that they came out to my house or even checked on me.

Once, I went into labor, my civilian coworker's husband came to get me to take me to the hospital, which was about 45 minutes away. At the hospital, I had my coworker's husband and coworker there for support. Later, some of my fellow soldiers came by to see and assist in the delivery of my baby, since I had been in labor all day. I had a complicated delivery and went in and out of consciousness, due to being exhausted and on medication. My friends recorded the delivery for my husband to see, but nothing takes the place of actually being there. Once the baby was delivered, everyone left, and I was alone for the first time with my newborn child. I was disheartened my husband missed the delivery of our first baby, and there was no way to tell him, except in a Red Cross message. I did not know if anyone sent a message until the hospital staff said they had sent one to him. All I could do now was wait for a phone call or letter to find out when he learned of his child's birth. My mother arrived the day after the baby was born and stayed for 10 days. After she had left, we were on our own again.

After my baby was born, one of my soldier friends asked me how I was handling being a new mother on my own. My friend also had a baby around the same time as me, but she had her civilian husband there to assist her with their baby's needs, and she still found the process to be overwhelming and difficult. My response to her was that you just have to do what you have to do. Although it was not easy, since you have to provide for your newborn with no one else there to help you. I was expected to be a soldier and a mom with no one to relieve me. There were nights I was on autopilot, especially when I went back to work and had early mornings with late night feedings. The scariest thing was going back to work and finding someone to take care of my newborn. You have to trust the person will be available at any given notice since as a soldier you have early mornings and late nights and can be deployed.

After I had gone back to work, I had less than 6 months left of my enlistment and had to make a decision to stay in the military. I thought about having to give my daughter to a relative, since my unit was preparing to deploy, and my husband was still deployed. At the time, I knew even if I changed duty stations, there was the possibility I would almost certainly be deployed. I also knew once my husband returned from his deployment he was eventually going to be attending Officer Basic Course for at least 3 months. Also, I thought about all the negativity from my command and the lack of support not just from one individual but instead from several of the individuals in the unit. The decision weighed on me, and I wished I could have made the decision with my spouse, but the topic was not something that could be decided in a quick phone call from overseas. I thought heavily on the decision to get out of the service and be a mother and a soldier's wife, instead of being the stellar soldier I once was.

Army Reserve (USAR) Father

I am a 46-year-old Captain in the United States Army Reserve. I am anything but a traditional reservist. I have served in the military for over 28 years and have deployed to both Iraq and Afghanistan after becoming a father. However, currently, I am serving on active duty on a stateside deployment, so I am able to go home at night, kiss my kids, read them bedtime stories and tuck them into bed. Although I am not separated from my family on this deployment, most of my deployments, I have been separated from them.

For instance, in 2003, I served as a Staff Sergeant in Iraq. When my reserve unit was mobilized, my wife was active duty and pregnant with our first daughter. On May 1, 2003, around the time George W. Bush gave his "Mission Accomplished" speech, I boarded a plane with my unit and deployed to Iraq. Within days of arriving in theater, I was patrolling the streets of Baghdad, Iraq, and was nervously awaiting the news of the birth of my first child.

My daughter was born on May 28, and my wife had to deliver our first child alone. I was not able to be present for the birth of our first daughter, nor was I able to witness the miracle of new life/entering into fatherhood. Instead, I was serving my country in a combat zone and did not even receive the news of my daughter's birth. Although I was sent a Red Cross message, it was delayed for 2 days.

I did not receive news of my daughter's birth until the new Company Commander and First Sergeant arrived in theater. I was given the news of my daughter's birth by a passing comment from my First Sergeant (1SG) when he asked what it was like to be a new father. Initially, his comment did not register, and then, it hit me. I asked for clarification and 1SG admitted he had forgotten to tell me he received the message 2 days prior. He then patted down his vest and pockets and retrieved a wrinkled, folded piece of paper and handed it to me. I opened it and read the Red Cross notice of my child's birth.

I was excited, confused, and pissed all at the same time. How could someone forget to relay this kind of news—especially for such a joyous occasion? I sat down and read the message over and over again until I finally put it away and had to resume my duties. I had to return to my position pulling security at my combat duty stationed. During security watch, I daydreamed of what it would be like to be a father and wondered what it was like for my wife to give birth to my daughter. Did it hurt? I had missed one of the most significant moments in the transition to fatherhood.

Although I would subsequently miss other moments, such as birthdays and anniversaries, missing my daughter's birth is the absence I most regret. This event would have a profound effect on me. The birth of my first child changed my marriage and signified my transition into fatherhood. It was no longer just the two of us, and my wife and I were responsible for a tiny human being.

I was angry I missed such a pivotal moment in my life, and my wife had to experience delivery alone. Unfortunately, our unit lost some soldiers who were killed in combat, which meant I was not able to go home to see my wife and daughter. I finally was able to return home 4 1/2 months later for mid-tour leave, where I was able to meet my daughter for the first time. I mourned the months I missed in her life and was surprised at how big she was.

I was only able to reunite with my family for 2 weeks and then had to return to a war zone. It wouldn't be until several months later that my deployment tour would be complete, and I would be able to be home for a longer duration.

After I returned home from Iraq, I still had to remain on active duty and was separated from my family for an additional four months. My wife and daughter were living several states away, so we did not see each other very often.

In 2005, I attended Officer Basic Course (OBC), which meant I was on active duty again and separated from my family for 4 months. Fortunately, during this separation, we were located in the same time zone, so it was easy to coordinate calling one another. In contrast, when I was deployed downrange, the time zone was at least 8hrs difference, so the time difference meant I had to plan carefully when I called home to ensure the least amount of disruption. It was important to me that their routines stayed on track.

From March 2008 to March 2009, I was deployed to the local Army base where I resided as a civilian. During this time period, my second child was born, and I finally had the opportunity to witness the miracle of birth. During this time, I was able to learn a lot about being a father and was able to participate more in my children's lives. During this stateside deployment, I was still able to drive my children to and from school and was present for my wife and children.

For me, returning to traditional reserve duty was less stressful on our household. The children got used to me having to work some weekends, but they knew I would be home at night. For them, it was just Dad going to work in a different uniform. Unfortunately, when I went back to my two weeks Annual Training (AT), it was a different matter. They would miss me and become emotional and cry. However, about the time I thought they would break, I was back home again.

From March 2010 to May 2011 and June 2011 to July 2012, I served two back-to-back tours in Afghanistan. During these deployments, we did a lot of Humanitarian Aid work to improve the lives of the local communities. Despite having the opportunity to help so many people, I couldn't help but notice helping others meant I was not there for my own family.

When I was deployed, my wife had to be a single geographical parent, and she had no assistance from her partner during overwhelming times. My wife managed to cope with this situation because she had no other choice. She had to become self-sufficient. She had to manage finances, pay the bills, walk the dogs, take care of the children, etc. I believed my absence affected my children since they often felt like a single parent was raising them.

When I returned home, we had to readjust family roles, as my children did not recognize me as an authority figure. I was now a different dad than the one who left them over a year before. My children did not know me and were upset with me for leaving them. They seemed to struggle with communicating this distress since they want you home but also fear you leaving them again. At times, my children would act out at home and would only respond to my wife's corrections. I had to learn how to reinsert myself back into my home life. I tried to have conversations with my daughters about why I was called away for the military. I believe eventually, my daughters will come to respect and understand my job and that freedom is not free.

After returning from 2 tours in Afghanistan, my children resented me and wanted me home. When I had to serve a month in Fort Erwin, California, my youngest daughter was at an age where she missed me more for this one month than she had ever missed me when I was in Afghanistan. While in Afghanistan, my daughter would talk to me on the phone, and my wife talked to her about me and would show her photos. In reality, it seemed like I was just some guy who visited once in a while. However, now, I was her daddy, *and she loved me equally as she did her mother. She was upset when I was leaving and kept asking why I couldn't get out of this duty assignment. I felt torn between my family and my duty.*

I didn't want to avoid this assignment since I would be helping other soldiers with training before they departed for their overseas assignment. My children's feelings of anger, abandonment, loss, etc. played themselves out again a year later when I again served for a month in Fort Polk, Louisiana. Despite all these conflicting feelings, I still feel it is an honor and privilege to serve in our military and to defend this nation. There is no greater responsibility than to serve our country in a time of war, even though I have had to make numerous personal sacrifices, including time away from my family.

Chapter 14

Future Directions

Melinda A. Thiam, David Hodson, and Karen L. Weis

Future Directions

To the best of our knowledge, this manuscript is the first of its kind to bring a consolidated multi-disciplinary and multi-service perspective on perinatal mental health in the military family. The completion of this manuscript was a multi-disciplinary effort between Army, Navy and Air Force health care providers, DoD civilian employees and perinatal experts such as Dr. Singly and Dr. Edwards willing to dedicate time and energy to increase awareness and provider education on perinatal mental health areas that affect the military family.

Obstetrics and Gynecology

The mission of the military health care is readiness, jointness and value. As the military aspires to increase and retain the number of women in the military as well as their top performing enlisted and officers, it is imperative that we offer a multi-disciplinary approach to behavioral and mental health care. It is clear that if mental health concerns are affecting any member of the family, it is affecting the readiness of the active duty member to perform to their best ability. We must continue to acknowledge and recognize mental health diagnoses and provide continuous and standardized support models across our military treatment centers and bases. As women's health care providers, we need to seek proactively education on topics of mental health in our population as well as promote the development and sustainment of case managers in the clinics who can see patients and families on the spot and provide them with resources and care. It is also important to recognize the perinatal mood and anxiety disorders and maintain continuity of care, especially in this age of 7-minute face-to-face time with our patients. Lastly, screening is not enough, but it is a start. We need to have programs in place for patients and their families that meet and exceed their needs.

Pediatrics/Family Medicine

Pediatricians and family medicine providers are key individuals to screen and assess the parent–infant relationship, and AAP Guidelines recommend screening for perinatal depression at prenatal and early well-child checks (AAP Guidelines, 2011; Talmi, Stafford, & Buchholz, 2009). Unfortunately, at this time, there is currently no specific DoD guideline about screening for parent mental health problems in pediatric well-child checks. However, in family medicine clinics, given providers are caring for the entire family, screening can be more easily implemented and has already started through programs like Army Child and Adolescent Behavioral Health Service.

Behavioral Health

It is imperative that research continues to provide insight and evidence-based approaches to the care and management of perinatal individuals and their families. Behavioral health providers, especially prescribing providers, need to be familiar with evidence-based treatments for perinatal mood and anxiety disorders and not fall into the trap that believes that lack of medication means no risk. As behavioral health providers, we are some of the key individuals to collaborate with primary care providers and empower primary care providers to assist in prescribing and treating mental health disorders.

Integrated Care

To date, the only published literature on the topic of military perinatal mental health comes from obstetrics, with several unpublished studies that have been presented at national conferences. We hope that this manuscript has inspired individuals to understand the plight of the military family and that this will be followed by more publication/national presentations on this topic. Many of the Perinatal Mental Health guidelines originate from organizations that have successfully created a periantal mental health service/recommendations. (COPE Guidelines, 2011; NICE Guidelines, 2014; Williams, 2014). We need more network providers able and willing to collaborate with providers within the Military Health system. With continued collaborated effort, we can make a difference for our military families. In the words of Michelle Obama and Jill Biden, "We can do this. In every community every day, we can find concrete ways to show our military families the respect and gratitude that each of us holds for them in our hearts" (The White House, 2011).

Key future goals include the following:

1. Recognize that perinatal mental health is essential in the treatment of the military family. Military family readiness translates to troop readiness

Taking care of military families at home, will help retain high-quality service members because they know that their families are being taken care of.

2. The collaboration of care: All disciplines, whether medicine, advanced practice nursing or therapists need to garner increased knowledge in the care and management of these perinatal individuals and to include safe treatment practices. These may include the management of psychotropic medications, and it would be advantageous to include PharmDs in the research process and clinical approach. The military can lead to the utilization of integrated health care, and this population can provide a segue for integrated health care to be a best practice rule rather than the exception.
    a. Standardize screening processes in primary care across obstetric/pediatrics and family medicine clinics and ensure there are a consultation process and case management support for primary care providers to refer positive screens.
    b. Empower behavioral health care providers to proactively consult with primary care providers and be able/willing to assist with treatment. Discuss proper informed consent and documentation to help decreased reluctance to treat due to legal liability concerns.
3. Networking with providers within the military health care system and surrounding community. Collaborate with organizations such as Postpartum Support International, Mothers of Preschoolers, National Fatherhood Initiative and educational/preparatory classes such as Bootcamp for New Dads and Boot Camp for New Moms.
4. Promotion of needs of military mothers and fathers. Continue to develop programs such as M-O-M-S™ program in antenatal care, as well as programs like mother–infant dyadic group therapy and support groups for new mothers and new fathers that can be implemented in military clinics across the DoD.

References

American Academy of Pediatrics. (2011). *Policy Statement: Screening for Postpartum Depression at Well-Child Visits*. LA Best Babies Network. (Accessed on December 2015). Retrieved from https://laperinatalmentalhealth.files.wordpress.com/2010/06/screeening-at-well-child-visits.pdf

BC Reproductive Mental Health Program. (2006). *Addressing Perinatal Depression: A Framework for BC's Health Authorities*. British Columbia, Canada: BC Women's Hospital & Health Centre, and Agency of the Provincial Health Services Authority.

BeyondBlue. (2011). Clinical Practice Guidelines (COPE): Depression and related disorders—Anxiety, bipolar disorder and puerperal psychosis—in the perinatal period: A guideline for primary care health professionals. Australian Government: National Health and Medical Research Counsel. Retrieved from www.beyondblue.org.au

National Institute of Health and Care Excellence (NICE). (2014). Antenatal and postnatal mental health: Clinical management and service guidelines. *Clinical Guideline*, December 17, 2014. Retrieved from www.Nice.org.uk/guidance/cg192

Talmi, A., Stafford, B., & Buchholz, M. (May, 2009). Providing perinatal mental health services in pediatric primary care. *Zero to Three, 29*(5), 10–16.

The White House. (2011). *Strengthening Our Military Families: Meeting America's Commitment.* Office of the Press Secretary. Thewhitehouse.gov Issues and Releases. Retrieved from www.whitehouse.gov, Keywords, Military families.

Williams, J. (2014). Best practice guidelines for mental health disorders in the perinatal period. *BC Mental Health.* Retrieved from www.perinatalservicesbc.ca/health-professionals/guidelines-standards/maternal (Accessed on 24 January, 2016).

Appendix

Body Image and Maternal Mental Health

Sharon Gerdes and Melinda A. Thiam

Overview

In Westernized society, body image is a critical aspect of a woman's identity, self-perception and self-esteem. Body image is conceptualized as one's internal perception of his or her outer appearance (Watson, Fuller-Tyszkiewicz, Broadbent, & Skouteris, 2015). Body image *disturbance* develops from the belief that one's appearance does not align with a desired or idealized body shape or size (Watson et al., 2015). Body image in pregnancy is dependent on how a woman is able to accept her changing size and body shape. Poor body image and body dissatisfaction are correlated with increased risk of perinatal mood and anxiety disorders in the postpartum period (Watson et al., 2015).

Body Image in the Military

Women's expectations and beliefs about their body, childbirth, and becoming a mother are strongly influenced by public, private and professional beliefs around birth and parenting (Roth et al., 2012). Given such, the cultural influence of military lifestyle can affect body image and subsequently influence mental health in pregnancy and postpartum.

All military services have stringent height and weight requirements to remain in service, and military mothers may be more likely than their civilian cohorts to enter pregnancy with a healthy weight and body composition. However, military women have different body types, and maintaining body weight and body fat composition requirements can be challenging (Smith, 2014). Service members who do not meet these standards are "flagged," meaning they can't go to military schools, get promoted, receive awards, and they are at risk for involuntary separation from military service. Military women have been found in studies to display increased amounts of disordered eating and maladaptive exercise behaviors. In one study, over 50% of female service members admitted that they exercised to control weight instead of doing so for fitness or general health reasons (Lauder et al., 1999).

Although all branches of military service wave height and weight standards during pregnancy, women typically have a 6-month postpartum period to return to pre-pregnancy body weight and fitness standards. For women who are already struggling with body image, the changes in weight and body fat contact that occur in pregnancy can lead to disordered eating patterns or precipitate an eating disorder. Even when all goes well, pregnancy and the postpartum period is a stressful time for a woman, with adjustments to family life, reduced sleep, and the stresses of caring for a newborn. Add to that the challenges of returning to pre-pregnancy weight, regardless of the reason—health, vanity or career—and it becomes clear that women need to find ways to achieve and maintain a healthy weight throughout the perinatal period without adding additional stress to their lives.

Biopsychosocial Factors that Contribute to Body Image

There are many factors that contribute to body image, especially as it relates to the pregnancy and postpartum period. In the following sections, we will address the biopsychosocial predisposing factors that contribute to development of a woman's body image. In particular, we will discuss factors that contribute to difficulties maintaining a healthy weight, or losing body weight in postpartum period (Karasu & Karasu, 2010). Body weight and body composition influence body image. In turn, body image in the transition to motherhood has a significant effect on a new mother's psychological health (Lacoursiere, Baksh, Bloebaum, & Varner, 2006).

Biological

Pre-Pregnancy Weight

Many women with body dissatisfaction during pregnancy often had body dissatisfaction prior to pregnancy (Watson et al., 2015). In the general population, there is a positive correlation between being overweight/obesity and increased likelihood of depression in women. Additionally, negative body image and overweight or obese status prior to pregnancy is predictive of developing depression postpartum (LaCoursiere, Barrett-Connor, O'Hara, Hutton, & Varner, 2010; Lacoursiere, Baksh, et al., 2010). In military women, those who struggle with maintaining body composition standards before pregnancy may struggle with negative self-image, experience body dissatisfaction, and participate in disordered eating in the postpartum period. When a military servicewoman becomes pregnant, this is one time in her career that body weight/composition standards are waived.

Weight Gain in Pregnancy

Despite health professional guidelines, many women gain more than the recommended amount of body weight during pregnancy, which can contribute to body dissatisfaction and negative body image (Siega-Riz et al., 2010). Like the civilian population, military women may also gain more weight than recommended, but unlike civilian cohort, military women have increased pressure for rapid weight loss postpartum. Although it takes them 9 months to gain all the weight, military women only have 6 months to return to normal weight.

Weight Loss Postpartum

The postpartum period is marked by preoccupation with returning to pre-pregnancy weight (Carwell & Spatz, 2011). Over 40% of new mothers report being dissatisfied in the postpartum period (Astrachan-Fletcher, Veldhuis, Lively, Fowler, & Marcks, 2008). Culturally, "getting your body back" after pregnancy has been the societal expectation for new mothers (Bedor &Tajima, 2012); it is a *requirement* for military mothers. Studies show that women who do not achieve their pre-pregnancy weight by 1 year postpartum are unlikely to ever return to pre-pregnancy weight. Military women who do not meet body weight standards will have body fat measured via a tape-measure. While many military women meet body fat standards despite being overweight, this is dependent on the individual who performs the body composition test. Measurement can vary depending on administrator. Variation in body composition measurements can mean sometimes women may pass body fat standards, but other times, despite absence of weight/body composition changes, are out of military standards.

History of Prior Eating Disorders

Approximately 10 million females in the United States are currently living with Anorexia or Bulimia Nervosa, and an additional 25 million people are struggling with Binge Eating Disorder (Astrachan-Fletcher et al., 2008; Carwell & Spatz, 2011). In the military, different studies found that 8% of military women met the criteria for an eating disorder, yet only 2% of women meeting criteria were actually diagnosed with an eating disorder (Manos, Carlton, & Kim, 2011).

When women with a current eating disorder or a history of one become pregnant, their underlying body image concerns and relationship with food and body weight resurface as they experience the weight gain and body changes that occur with pregnancy. Studies have found that while body satisfaction, eating disturbances, and overall eating disorder symptoms improve during pregnancy, eating disorders frequently resurface and actually may worsen in the postpartum period (Carwell & Spatz, 2011).

Exercise and Fitness

Exercise can counteract body dissatisfaction and promote body acceptance, especially during and after pregnancy. A high amount of exercise in pregnancy (defined as at least 90 minutes per week) was correlated with increased body satisfaction at 15- to 22-week gestation compared to a minimal amount of exercise (Boscaglia, Skouteris, & Wertheim, 2003). Physical activity throughout the course of pregnancy improves both physical and psychological health, and some studies confirm that consistent exercise in the pre-pregnancy period may prevent the occurrence of depressive symptoms in early pregnancy (Downs, DiNallo, & Kirner, 2008).

Military women may particularly struggle with exercise in the postpartum period, and often struggle with training the correct way to pass their military service specific fitness test within 6 months postpartum (Boyle, 2014). The pressure to return to pre-baby fitness levels can be both helpful as well as potentially harmful. While the expectation for fitness may lead military mothers to be more active during pregnancy and postpartum, it can also create a double-edged sword, and military women may use exercises as a purging method as part of disordered eating.

Stress Hormones/Sleep Deprivation

Chronic exposure to stress and high cortisol levels during pregnancy can increase the likelihood of high gestational weight gain, weight retention in postpartum, and a higher likelihood of obesity later in life (Siega-Riz et al., 2010). Women who felt depressed, distressed or anxious during pregnancy had a higher postpartum weight retention at both 6 and 18 months (Pedersen et al., 2011). Support groups for new mothers might assist in easing the stress of adjustment to motherhood, and assistance with childcare might also reduce stress levels. Specific stress factors for military families include return to active duty, meeting physical fitness and weight targets postpartum, and the deployment of the spouse.

Sleep

Another factor affecting weight management is sleep. One study showed a link between shorter sleep duration and obesity (Hill et al., 2013). At 6 months postpartum, women who slept 5 hours or less per day showed significantly greater rates of substantial postpartum weight retention than women who slept 6, 7 or 8 or more hours per day. The authors suggest that interventions to attain optimal maternal sleep should be included as part of a strategy to prevent postpartum obesity (Gunderson et al., 2008). Another study examined sleep duration at 3 and 12 months, and found an association between less than 5 hours of sleep and excess weight retention.

Psychological

Numerous psychological factors contribute to body image. A mother's self-esteem and mental health, as well as her prior eating behaviors and beliefs about food, can increase likelihood of increased gestational weight gain (Hill et al., 2013). Women with high depressive symptoms in pregnancy show high trait anxiety, low self-esteem, and less tolerance to stress (Hill et al., 2013). Mothers with poor coping skills have increased likelihood of increased gestational weight gain and poorer body dissatisfaction.

Eating Attitudes

Pregnancy can affect eating behaviors as it presents women with an opportunity to "eat for two" and to abandon diet plans and enjoy body weight and changes for the health of their baby (Scloim et al., 2013). Both individuals who overindulge or excessively restrict have increased likelihood of greater gestational weight gain (Scloim et al., 2013). Individual beliefs about eating prior to pregnancy will influence what she believes about a healthy diet in pregnancy and postpartum. Some women are emotional eaters and may turn to food for comfort, stress relief or as a reward. The extent to which eating becomes emotional may have a strong effect on weight management. In one study, 27% of women displayed psychological and behavioral features associated with an eating disorder during the perinatal period (Easter et al., 2013).

Dyadic

Relation with Infant

A mother's body image and eating habits can lead to physical and psychological consequences for her child (Astrachan-Fletcher et al., 2008). Women with disordered eating and body image concerns may be overly concerned with their child's weight and body shape (Astrachan-Fletcher et al., 2008). Mothers with disordered eating may utilize restrictive feeding behaviors with their children, sometimes starting as early as breastfeeding (Astrachan-Fletcher et al., 2008). Mothers with disordered eating are more likely to bottle feed, less likely to breastfeed, and may fail to recognize their child's cues while eating (Astrachan-Fletcher et al., 2008). Other studies have found that maternal disinhibition, body dissatisfaction, hunger, BMI, and bulimic symptoms in the first month of an infant's life predict that the child has an increased chance of engaging in secretive eating behaviors. Maternal restraint predicts that the child may engage in overeating by age 5 (Astrachan-Fletcher et al., 2008).

Relationship with Partner

Women with poor marital/partner relationships, less social support, may be more prone to postpartum depression and concurrent weight management issues (Hill et al., 2013). A woman's body image can influence marital satisfaction and likelihood of returning to marital intimacy (Hill et al., 2013) or she may struggle with weight/body image concern due to emotional abuse or negative evaluation by her partner (Scott, 2009).

Family of Origin

Body image of maternal and attachment figures growing up will influence how a woman develops a body image as well as her sense of being in control/out of control of body weight and eating. Mothers who hold personal concerns about their own weight often believe that restricting and monitoring their child's intake will lead to healthy eating habits (Brown, 2014). Additionally, a mother has significant influence on her daughter's body image, and how a mother treats and refers to her body can affect how her daughter experiences her body (Zeilinger, 2015). In some studies, as many as 1 in 4 children have engaged in some type of dieting behavior by age 7 (Zeilinger, 2015), and a history of dieting behavior in childhood will predispose a woman to disordered eating and dieting behaviors as an adult.

Group Identity and Social Roles

Active Duty Mothers

Active duty mothers likely have had a high fitness level prior to pregnancy. Depending on the pregnancy and type of delivery, the inability to return to prior fitness levels may impact how peers see her, and how she sees herself. Active duty mothers may push themselves to hurry back to pre-baby weight, and feel pressure by peers and military commands to lose all excess weight rapidly. Active duty mothers who struggle with body composition are often at risk of this interfering with career progression. Even if they are not flagged, if they are seen as overweight—even if technically meeting body fat standards, they may be socially ostracized by peers who view them negatively. They may also be subjected to potential negative reactions from commanders who are very adamant about strict military appearance.

Military Spouse

Given military emphasis on lean body frame, military spouses may feel obligated to likewise have a fit and trim appearance. If they do not meet this expectation, they may fear they will be judged negatively by the military community or an active duty spouse. They may feel that their husband is comparing them to active duty women (usually those who are not mothers) who are able to keep fit and trim.

Societal

In Westernized society, we associate thin individuals with having self-discipline and hard work, while fatness is often assumed to be secondary to gluttony and lack of willpower (Bedor & Tajima, 2012). While society may give permission for mothers to gain weight during pregnancy, this attitude rapidly shifts in the postpartum period. The media plays a powerful role in shaping, framing and proliferation of certain body image ideologies (Roth, Homer & Fenwick, 2012). Such cultural expectation can be seen by evaluating how celebrity pregnancies are perceived in the media. Body changes associated with pregnancy may be seen as unnatural and unhealthy, while returning to one's pre-pregnancy body shape is approached in a similar fashion as recovering from illness (Roth et al., 2012). Celebrity role models and their journey through pregnancy have been widely scrutinized in magazines and social media (Bedor &Tajima, 2012; Roth et al., 2012). Celebrities who have ready access to trainers, chefs and childcare often bounce back to pre-pregnancy weight in 6 weeks. This creates pressure on other women to achieve a similar quick return to pre-pregnancy weight, which may be unrealistic for women with modest financial resources. Using celebrity mothers as role models, advertisers and marketers can prey on the desires and insecurities of women, creating unrealistic societal expectations.

Cultural

There is a positive association between maternal beliefs, well-being and pregnancy outcomes. However, the pressure to achieve and maintain slimness is prevalent and pervasive within Western cultures where pressure to achieve and maintain slimness abound. One study that compared new mothers in the United Kingdom and Israel found lower body satisfaction in mothers in Israel. The authors suggest that the stress of living in a combat zone might contribute to negative body image. The stress of living in a combat zone during pregnancy, or even having a spouse deployed to a combat zone during pregnancy, might negatively affect body image.

Summary

Numerous factors affect body image for the active duty military woman and the military spouse. Excessive weight gain during pregnancy, as well as social and societal factors, can all exert a negative effect on body image. It is important to recognize the existence of negative body image and body dissatisfaction amongst military women in general, and understand how body image can be impacted by pregnancy. Military and dependent mothers struggling with perinatal mood or anxiety disorders should be evaluated for presence of negative body image and assessed for potential eating disorder symptoms.

References

Astrachan-Fletcher, E., Veldhuis, C., Lively, N., Fowler, C., & Marcks, B. (2008). The reciprocal effects of eating disorders and the postpartum period: A review of the literature and recommendations for clinical care. *Journal of Women's Health, 17*(2), 227–239.

Bedor, E., & Tajima, A. (2012). No fat moms! Celebrity mother's weight-loss narratives in people magazine. Paper presented at the annual meeting of the International Communication Association, TBA, Boston, MA, May 25, 2011

Boscaglia, N., Skouteris, H., & Wertheim, E. (2003). Changes in body image satisfaction during pregnancy: A comparison of high exercising and low exercising women. *Australian and New Zealand Journal of Obstetrics and Gynaecology, 43*(1), 41–45. doi: 10.1046/j.0004-8666.2003.00016.x

Boyle, A. (2014). New Mothers May Need Counseling, Training to Pass Postpartum Military Fitness Test. U.S. Medicine: The Voice of Federal Medicine. Retrieved from www.usmedicine.com

Brown, A. (2014). Maternal restraint and external eating behaviour are associated with formula use or shorter breastfeeding duration. *Appetite, 76*, 30–35.

Carwell, M., & Spatz, D. (2011). Eating disorders and breastfeeding. *Maternal Child Nursing, 36*(2), 112–117.

Downs, D., DiNallo, J., & Kirner, T. (2008). Determinants of pregnancy and postpartum depression: Prospective influences of depressive symptoms, body image satisfaction, and exercise behavior. *Annuals of Behavioral Medicine, 36*, 54–63.

Easter, A., Bye, A., Taborelli, E., Corifield, F., Schmidt, U., Treasure, J., & Micali, Nadia. (2013). Recognizing the symptoms: How common are eating disorders in pregnancy? *European Eating Disorders, 21*, 340–344.

Gunderson, E. P., Rifas-Shiman, S. L., Oken, E., Rich-Edwards, J. W., Kleinman, K. P., Taveras, E. M., & Gillman, M. W. (2008). Association of fewer hours of sleep at 6 months postpartum with substantial weight retention at 1 year postpartum. *American Journal of Epidemiology, 167*(2), 178–187. doi:10.1093/aje/kwm298

Hill, B., Skouteris, H., McCabe, M., Milgrom, J., Kent, B., Herring, S., . . . MCommerce. (2013). A conceptual model of psychosocial risk and protective factors for excessive gestational weight gain. *Midwifery, 29*, 110–114.

Karasu, S. R., & Karasu, T. B. (2010). *The Gravity of Weight: A Clinical Guide to Weight Loss and Maintenance* (1st ed.). Washington, DC: American Psychiatric Pub.

Lacoursiere, D. Y., Baksh, L., Bloebaum, L., & Varner, M. W. (2006). Maternal body mass index and self-reported postpartum depressive symptoms. *Maternal Child Health Journal, 10*(4), 385–390. doi:10.1007/s10995-006-0075-1

LaCoursiere, D. Y., Barrett-Connor, E., O'Hara, M. W., Hutton, A., & Varner, M. W. (2010). The association between prepregnancy obesity and screening positive for postpartum depression. *BJOG, 117*(8), 1011–1018. doi:10.1111/j.1471-0528.2010.02569.x

Lauder, T., Williams, M., Campbell, C., Davis, G., & Sherman, R. (1999). Abnormal eating behaviors in military women. *Medicine & Science in Sports and Exercise, 31*(9), 1265–1271.

Manos, G., Carlton, J., & Kim, A. (2011). Chapter 28: Eating disorders. In C. Ritchie (Ed.), *Combat and Operational Behavioral Health*. Fort Sam Houston, TX: Office of the Surgeon General, Department of the Army & Army Medical Department Center and School. Retrieved from www.cs.amedd.army.mil/borden/

Milgrom, J., Skouteris, H., Worotniuk, T., Henwood, A., & Bruce, L. (2012). The association between ante- and postnatal depressive symptoms and obesity in both mother and child: A systematic review of the literature. *Women's Health Issues, 22*(3), e319–e328.

Pedersen, P., Baker, J. L., Henriksen, T. B., Lissner, L., Heitmann, B. L., Sørensen, T. I., & Nohr, E. A. (2011). Influence of psychosocial factors on postpartum weight retention. *Obesity (Silver Spring), 19*(3), 639–646. doi:10.1038/oby.2010.1752

Roth, H., Homer, C., & Fenwick, J. (2012). Bouncing back: How Australia's leading women's magazines portray the postpartum "body". *Women and Birth, 25*, 128–124.

Scloim, N., Hetherington, M., Rudolf, M., & Feltbower, R. (2013). Relationship between body mass index and women's body image, self-esteem and eating behaviors in pregnancy: A cross-cultural study. *Journal of Health Psychology, 20*(4), 13–26. doi: 10.1177/1359105313502568.

Scott, B. (2009). Maternal Trauma and Body Image Attitudes during Pregnancy. Dissertation for Master of science in Psychology, Oklahoma State University, Stillwater, OK.

Siega-Riz, A. M., Herring, A. H., Carrier, K., Evenson, K. R., Dole, N., & Deierlein, A. (2010). Sociodemographic, perinatal, behavioral, and psychosocial predictors of weight retention at 3 and 12 months postpartum. *Obesity (Silver Spring), 18*(10), 1996–2003. doi:10.1038/oby.2009.458

Smith, S. (2014). An Incredible Number of Women in the Military Battle Eating Disorders. Care 2. 27 February, 2014. Retrieved from www.care2.com

Watson, B., Fuller-Tyszkiewicz, M., Broadbent, J., & Skouteris, H. (2015). The meaning of body image experiences during the perinatal period: A systematic review of the qualitative literature. *Body Image, 14*, 102–113.

Zeilinger, J. (2015). How Mothers Shape Their Daughter's Body Image. *Identities.Mic* Retrieved from www.mic.com

Index

Note: Page numbers in *italics* indicate tables and figures.

For Product Safety Concerns and Information please contact our EU
representative GPSR@taylorandfrancis.com
Taylor & Francis Verlag GmbH, Kaufingerstraße 24, 80331 München, Germany

www.ingramcontent.com/pod-product-compliance
Ingram Content Group UK Ltd.
Pitfield, Milton Keynes, MK11 3LW, UK
UKHW022204190926
475702UK00003B/191

* 9 7 8 1 1 3 8 9 2 4 7 7 2 *